MEMBERSHIP PRIMARY CARE

D1620625

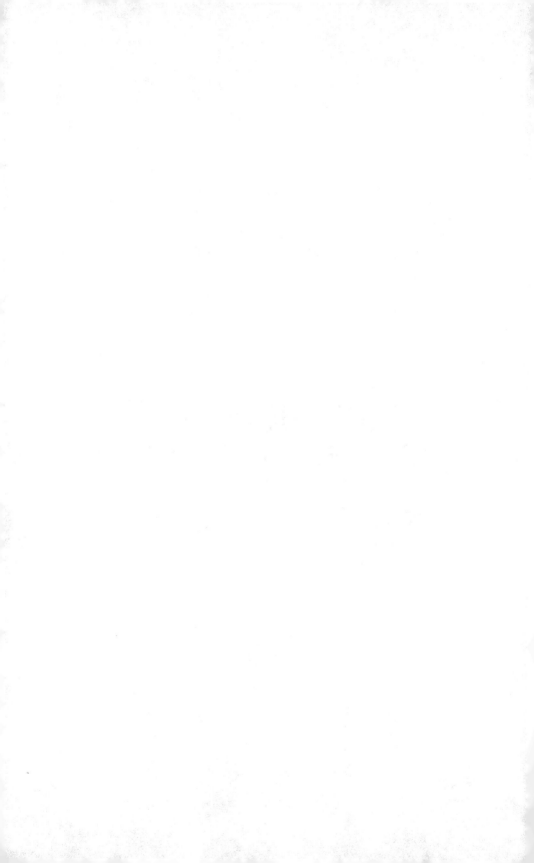

ROBERT T. BAILEY, PHARMD, MD

MEMBERSHIP PRIMARY CARE:

Transforming Family Medicine is Key to Health Care Reform

XULON PRESS ELITE

Xulon Press Elite
2301 Lucien Way #415
Maitland, FL 32751
407.339.4217
www.xulonpress.com

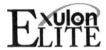

© 2021 by Robert T. Bailey, PharmD, MD

All rights reserved solely by the author. The author guarantees all contents are original and do not infringe upon the legal rights of any other person or work. No part of this book may be reproduced in any form without the permission of the author. The views expressed in this book are not necessarily those of the publisher.

Due to the changing nature of the Internet, if there are any web addresses, links, or URLs included in this manuscript, these may have been altered and may no longer be accessible. The views and opinions shared in this book belong solely to the author and do not necessarily reflect those of the publisher. The publisher therefore disclaims responsibility for the views or opinions expressed within the work.

Unless otherwise indicated, Scripture quotations taken from New Life Version (NLV). Copyright © 1969 by Christian Literature International.

Scripture quotations taken from the King James Version (KJV) – *public domain*.

Scripture quotations taken from the Holy Bible, New International Version (NIV). Copyright © 1973, 1978, 1984, 2011 by Biblica, Inc.™. Used by permission. All rights reserved.

Cover Illustration: "The Difficult Case," by Nathan Greene, © 2001, All Rights Reserved, Used by Permission. www.nathangreene.com

Library of Congress Control Number: 2021909381

Paperback ISBN-13: 978-1-6628-1843-1
Ebook ISBN-13: 978-1-6628-1844-8

Patient Reviews

I am an eye doctor in Scottsdale, and I have many opportunities to know the primary care physicians in my area. I had the chance to see quite a few of Dr. Bailey's patients, and they all rave about his care. Subsequently, having gotten to know Dr. Bailey, I was so impressed that I switched to have him become my doctor. He is kind, patient, and incredibly thorough. His "routine" physical includes so many valuable assessments (including nutritional blood work) that it takes an hour to review them, and he does so methodically. Kathy, who runs his office, is always pleasant and has great follow-through. Having Dr. Bailey as my doctor is like taking a step back in time. While his diagnostic work is very current, well-researched, and cutting edge, his demeanor takes me back to a time when doctors took more time with patients and were interested in the total patient. I recommend him highly and without any reservation.

—Dr. Stephen C.

I had a very highly valued session with Dr. Bailey. I have never experienced this level of professionalism, care, and help from a health care professional. Dr. Bailey is on the cutting edge of helping his patients lower their risk factors for disease, instead of just treating the symptoms of disease until they manifest themselves into a difficult, if not life-threatening, situation. Dr. Bailey, in my view, represents the doctor of the future and probably the last hope for really dealing with the health care crisis in an effective and brilliant manner. I feel privileged to have the honor of being one of his patients.

—**Gary S.**

Excellent and personalized care. Dr. Bailey listens closely and spends the time to diagnose properly. Thank you, Dr. Bailey.

—**David E.**

The entire health care team at Dr. Bailey's medical facility should be commended for their performance during my recent annual physical. Each person contributed to the overall experience. I am always concerned about any abnormalities found, but Dr. Bailey puts it all in perspective, and his support team members, from the front desk to the medical assistant, are professionals and make me feel like I am special.

—**Dennis M.**

I felt so relieved! You have started me on a new journey to health. You *listened* and came up with a *plan* to address my concerns. I feel for the first time that there was someone special that would use all his knowledge, along with his team, to make me a healthier and happier person. I look forward to a long and successful friendship in health.

—**Margaret J.**

Doc is always full of info to help to get results in what he does and what I must do. I feel that he explains everything in depth, and it is easy to understand and easy for me to ask questions.

—Frieda S.

Close, personal attention intending to substantially extend my lifespan. Membership has its privileges, but it's the medical team that does the research and develops my unique and effective plan to ensure good health.

—Dennis N.

As usual, the visit was thorough and informative. Dr. Bailey took the time to explain in detail the results of my tests, tweaked my medication and suggested ways to improve my health in the future. I was the last appointment of the day, and I'm sure if I had more questions Dr. Bailey would have stayed until 8:00 p.m. answering them.

—Henry V.

As I have repeatedly told my wife, this is the best medical care that I have ever experienced.

—Thomas H.

It's the "prevent defense" that I love—testing for possibilities, addressing any weaknesses, his teams, of which I am a member—this is a dream medical situation, and I thank God someone told me about Bailey Family Medical Care (www.baileyfamilymedical-care.com) a number of years ago. It has only become better with the restructuring, so my husband is now enjoying the same relationship. We have confidence!

—Carla H.

Dr. Bailey is a very caring doctor and takes the time to know you as a person.

—Kathy B.

Dedication

I dedicate this book and express my gratitude to my Lord and Savior Jesus Christ, who is the way, the truth, and the life, and who has restored me to right standing with my loving Heavenly Father God, now and for eternity. He said Himself that He is written of in the volume or entirety of the Book (Old and New Testament of the Bible). It is in Him that I live, move, and have my being. He is the Alpha and the Omega, the beginning and the end, the bright Morningstar, the Word of God, the only begotten Son of our Heavenly Father, the perfect sacrificial lamb, who died for the sins of the world, the returning Lion of the tribe of Judah, Christ Jesus, the chief cornerstone whom the builders rejected, and the one who was raised from the dead and who ascended into Heaven, where He sits on the right hand of the Father until His enemies are made His footstool.

He stands at the door of our hearts and knocks, and if we will open the door, He will come in and eat and have fellowship with us. He will never leave or forsake us. There is nowhere we can go and no condition so dire that we can hide from Him. He will find us even in our worst condition. He is a friend of the sinner and our friend. Though our sins be like scarlet, Jesus will wash us whiter than snow. He has promised us eternal life if we will ask Him and repent and follow His teachings. I pray this will come to pass for me and everyone that reads this book.

I also dedicate this book to my wonderful parents, Bob (Robert, Sr.) and Lessie Rhoad Bailey, of North Charleston, South Carolina, who passed along to me and my older sister, Mary Shannon, their capacity for using their high intellect. They modeled an integrous life dedicated to faith, family, and freedom, and their experiences and examples have motivated us well into our adult years. Mom and Dad stood behind me and supported me in my decision to go to medical school at the mature age of thirty-five. My dad was blessed to have graduated from the US Naval Academy in 1939 with a BS in metallurgic engineering. Mom, who grew up in rural South Carolina, was awarded a BS in biology from Winthrop College in 1944, managing to graduate from college in the first half the twentieth century. She worked so she could pay her own tuition and room and board. This was not such an easy accomplishment for a woman from rural South Carolina in those days.

They were among the pillars of their community, and Dad was a founding member of the North Charleston Methodist Church. He actually broke ground on the church building and the educational buildings in November 1954. He served in many lay capacities in the church, including on the board of directors, and he headed up most of the church committees for many years. He was a role model to many of the younger men in the church. He was faithful in his attendance and as a tither and giver.

Poem by Robert T. Bailey on Membership Primary Care

A Membership Primary Care Physician is a Doctor Who Knows You by Your First Name.

A Doctor Who Knows Your Current Medical History and Medical Problems.

A Doctor Who Knows All the Medications and Supplements You Take.

A Doctor Who Knows All the Other Physicians You See, and Retrieves Their Office Notes to Carefully Review on an Ongoing Basis.

A Doctor Who Tracks Down All Your Test Results and Follows Up with You in a Timely Manner.

A Doctor Who Is Able to Diagnose, Treat, and Manage Most of Your Diseases and Medications.

A Doctor Who Is Interested in Your Health, not Just Your Illnesses.

A Doctor Who Makes Sure Your Healthcare Is Not Directed nor Dictated by a Third-Party Health Insurance Company.

A Membership Doctor is Not *Just* Secondary Care, or Follow Up Care, or Urgent Care, but A Doctor Who Is Your Primary Care Doctor for Life.

SCRIPTURES

Scripture quotes in this book are taken from the New Living Translation (NLV) the King James Version (KJV).

> "My people are destroyed for lack of knowledge. Because you have rejected knowledge, I also will reject you from being priest for Me; Because you have forgotten the law of your God, I also will forget your children" (Hosea 4:6, NLV).

> "And the very God of peace sanctify you wholly; and I pray God your whole spirit and soul and body be preserved blameless unto the coming of our Lord Jesus Christ" (1 Thess. 5:23, KJV).

Notable Quotes on Courage Needed to Challenge the Status Quo in Medicine

"One man with courage makes a majority"
(Andrew Jackson).

"The courage we desire, and prize is not the courage to die decently but to live manfully"
(Thomas Carlyle).

"The hottest places in Hell are reserved for those who, in a time of great moral crisis, maintain their neutrality"
(Dante).

"Courage is defined as 'grace under pressure'"
(Ernest Hemingway).

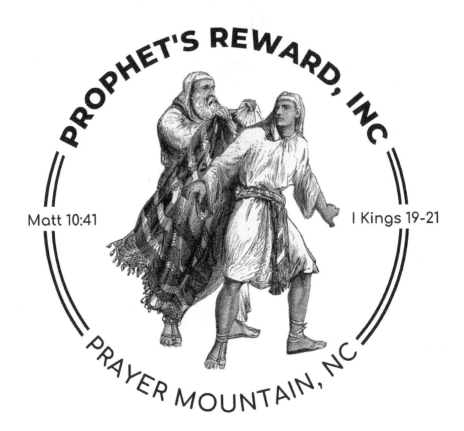

Mission Statement: Prophet's Reward, Inc.

Prophet's Reward is a nonprofit corporation organized and existing under the laws of the State of North Carolina. Dr. Bailey is the organization's president. It was organized for the purposes of advancing and promoting the worship and the fellowship of God through the provision and development of a facility on Prayer Mountain, in Moravian Falls, NC. The facility will be used for study of the Bible, as well as meditation and reflection on the Holy Scriptures. We believe that the Bible is the revealed Word of God, the teaching and furthering of the Gospel of our Lord and Savior Jesus Christ. Prophet Reward's mission is to provide the public with both the physical facilities and scholarly materials for various methods of education, including needed medical research, reform, the advancement of whole person medicine and clearer understanding of the Word of God, both written and prophetically spoken. Prophet's Reward exists to bring health, healing, and wholeness to individuals by natural, scientific, and divine supernatural methods. Clarifying and promoting the role of the integrated family physician, who can spend the needed time with his or her patients, is a primary mission of reform detailed in *Membership Primary Care*.

Prophet's Reward, Inc. also strives to provide a flexible educational ministry, which provides spiritual training and Christian development that will benefit those that the company members encounter, to equip them to win souls for Jesus Christ and develop mature followers of His teachings. The purposes of the company shall be missionary in spirit, extending the Gospel using the company property and of various developed business platforms for the use of our neighbors, our community, and to the entire world. www.prophetsreward.org

The Moravians believed in influencing society for the glory of God. Based in Germany, they were the first Christians to send missionaries out into the world, including to the Eastern United States. Prior to the American Revolutionary War, they ministered not only to white settlers but natives and slaves. In honor of their purchase and settlement of a 100,000-acre tract of land in North Carolina, called Wachovia, and to the small but special town of Moravian Falls, North Carolina named after them, and to their hundred years of continuous intercessory prayer during the settlement of Moravian Falls, NC, the Lord directed Johanna and me to establish Prophet's Reward, Inc., on Prayer Mountain, in Moravian Falls.

John Wesley founded the Methodist Church, but it was the Moravians who profoundly influenced him on one of his trips from Europe back to the United States. The ship he was traveling on sailed into a violent storm one night, and the passengers were sure the ship would sink. John Wesley observed the calmness and peace of the Moravians—men, women, and children—as they worshipped God. Having survived the storm, Wesley sought to learn of the beliefs and the lifestyle of the Moravians, and through this fellowship, he formed much of his working theology, and he received the baptism of the Holy Spirit that empowered his ministry in the US and England.

Beginning in March 1739, traveling alone throughout England and the United States on horseback, Wesley began open-air preaching. Rather than speak about salvation through good works and righteous living, he began to preach about salvation through faith in Christ. It is said that Wesley road over 250,000 miles by horseback, preaching the Gospel of Jesus Christ. What I respect most about John Wesley is that he received strategies from Heaven for launching lay people into the ministry. John Wesley also believed in unity through diversity. He said, "Each of us is meant to be an original, but most of us die merely a copy." This accelerated the Methodist movement he started, and by 1830, Methodism had become the largest Christian denomination in the United States.

The Methodists became a major contributor to the Pentecostal movement 150 years later. The enthusiastic style of worship that characterizes Pentecostal church services today is reminiscent of early nineteenth-century Methodist revivals and camp meetings. They were called the "Shouting Methodist" in the early 19th century. The strict fundamentalist regulations imposed upon Pentecostal believers originate largely from the "Holiness" tradition, which was itself an outgrowth of John Wesley's Methodist beliefs of sanctification. Today, Pentecostalism is the fastest growing religious denomination in the world, with an estimated 500 million adherents.

Johanna and I purchased seventeen acres of pristine, anointed, wooded land on Prayer Mountain North Carolina in the fall of 2017. We did this in appreciation of the generational blessing of my father, Robert T. Bailey, Sr. (1917–2015); my grandfather, Gratton M. Bailey (1880–1952), both from Bluefield, Virginia; my great grandfather, Jesse Bailey, Jr. (1835–1901), from Tazwell County, Virginia; and of my great, great, great, great grandfather, Captain James Moore (1740–1786), of Abbs Valley, Virginia, who fought as a militia captain during the American Revolution at the 1781 Battle of Guilford Court House in North Carolina. When one looks due north from our property near the top of Prayer Mountain, Bluefield, Tazwell County and Abbs Valley, VA are hidden among the peaks and valleys of the Blue Ridge Mountains only about 133 miles away. In honor of these great men, we plan to develop a prayer and meditation garden and retreat center on Prayer Mountain to teach and foster a deeper understanding of the Word of God and provide a refuge and training facility for God's modern-day prophets and leaders.

An arm of Prophet's Reward, Inc., is dedicated to advancing truth, justice, and reform in our health care system, so our citizens can benefit from health, healing, and wholeness. I was ordained as a Christian minister of medicine in 1994. *Membership Primary Care* is our first publication in support of one the main missions of Prophet's Reward, Inc. Please pray that God will use it to help reform healthcare in our country and please be sure to visit our website at: www.prophetsreward.org.

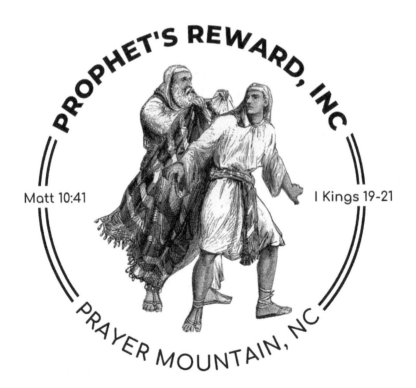

Table of Contents

Chapter 1	Demand for Family Physicians Is Great, but Not Without Challenges	1
Chapter 2	Why Is It Vital to Have an Independent Membership Family Physician?	12
Chapter 3	How to Identify a Family Physician who Is Personal, Compassionate, and Scientific	27
Chapter 4	What is a Membership-Based Family Medicine Practice Model?	35
Chapter 5	Expanding Availability of Membership Family Physicians Is the Key to Health Care Reform	39
Chapter 6	An Integrated Family Physician Is Essential in the Twenty-First Century to a Successful Membership Practice	51
Chapter 7	Heart Attacks and Strokes Are Preventable: The BaleDoneen Method Is a Premier Integrated Membership Practice	55
Chapter 8	Personalized Medical-Grade Nutritional Supplements Are Critical to Health and Wellness for Most Patients	62

Chapter 9	Faith and Medicine Are Compatible and Desirable and Can be Mixed with Sensitivity and Compassion	69
Chapter 10	Health Insurance Is not Health Care	75
Chapter 11	The COVID Debacle and the Medical Mafia	79
Chapter 12	Bailey Family Medical Care: Prototype for Membership Medicine	87

Foreword

I had the pleasure of meeting Dr. Robert Bailey in Atlanta, GA in 2015. As the Founder and Publisher of the emerging Direct Care industry's trade and professional resource, Concierge Medicine Today (CMT), I made a point of meeting many the doctors attending CMT's Concierge Medicine Forum that year. I felt an immediate drawing to Robert. It quickly became apparent as to why. We promptly settled into a deep discussion about the general state of the healthcare system, the meaning and value behind this important patient care movement, and the moral obligation of physicians as it moves forward. I found him to be highly knowledgeable, greatly insightful, deeply spiritual, and totally committed to his practice, his patients, the community he serves, and personally to his family and to the Lord. I found myself wishing that there were more doctors who were as knowledgeable and passionate as he about these things. Working in an influential trade publication and resource organization in the membership medicine movement, I have had the privilege of working with some brilliant physicians and great minds. As I came to know Robert better, I found that my initial impression of him was just scratching the surface of the depth of the man and seasoned clinician I have come to admire as a professional colleague and friend. With his vast experience and successful membership medicine practice, it is only proper that he write a book on behalf of this movement for its potential patients everywhere.

This book is important on many levels and is highly relevant to today's healthcare discussion. For the patient, it provides much needed information regarding what membership medicine is, how and why it developed, and the benefits of employing a personal physician advocate. Dr. Bailey also outlines what to look for when looking for a physician operating in this innovative model of healthcare delivery. He sets the bar high and meets it every day. Dr. Bailey is an advocate of integrative medicine, the blending of the best of western medicine while incorporating tried and proven complementary-alternative medicine for the purposes of preventing disease. Blending this approach with his deep and uncompromising Christian faith, you see the outcome is a physician who not only wants you to receive the best healthcare, but he also wants you whole: mind, body, soul, and spirit. 1 Corinthians 10:24 (NIV) states, "No one should seek their own good, but the good of others." Robert clearly demonstrates this through the insights shared in this book. He may not be Marcus Welby, MD, but he's close. Just ask his patients.

This book is riddled with facts and information that will give the reader understanding of how our healthcare system is currently structured, how it is failing us and how membership medicine and other direct care models of healthcare delivery can save lives, preserve resources, and help to achieve a healthier America. It is a subject about which he is both knowledgeable and passionate. You will see this as you begin your journey towards better health and a better healthcare system through learning what is contained herein. His conscience required that he help you to become a better-informed health care consumer and patient. His faith demanded it. We will all be the better for applying what we learn from this wise physician.

Enjoy and take lots of notes. You will want to share them with friends and family and remember them when you are looking for your next physician advocate.

J. Catherine Sykes
Founder and Publisher
Concierge Medicine Today
The Direct Primary Care Journal

Introduction

As we enter the third decade of the twenty-first century, the health care system in the United States needs massive reform. Health care is riddled with excessive costs and regulations. Doctors are burned out and leaving their once-great profession, family physicians most of all. Their doctor roles are being taken over by nurse practitioners and physician assistants practicing medicine by protocols and algorithms. In contrast, physicians with extensive years of education and training in college, medical school and residency and fellowship training programs, are slowly being replaced by nonphysicians with significantly less education and training. Their leadership desires that they be allowed to work independent of physician oversight and supervision. They often assume the role of the primary care physician, not so much through extensive years of education and practice experience in the laboratory of clinical medicine, but rather the brightest and best nurses leaving their great profession of nursing to practice medicine. With the large number of nurses going on to become nurse practitioners, this has left a shortage in nursing care and leadership in hospitals. This gap in available registered nurses is being filled with lesser trained nursing type individuals trying to take their place in hospitals. This results in the registered nurses being assigned too many patients to care for and thus patients often receive suboptimal nursing care.

As we move into the future, the anticipated physician shortage grows worse with each passing year because of the ineffective leadership in medicine and refusal to fix the broken parts and replace the missing pieces of our profession. The largest health care crisis in America is *not* that every man, woman, and child is not insured (though the creators of Obamacare seemed to think it was) it's that primary care physicians, the great diagnosticians and patient educators, are becoming an endangered species. Very few have recognized that having a manageable number of patients and enough time to spend with each patient are critical to making a sizable and lasting difference in clinical outcomes and patient satisfaction. The profession of medicine has made the critical error of utilizing the primary care physician as a high-volume triage agent—"feeders" for specialists and hospital systems—rather than the health care navigator for the patient throughout their medical journey and the hub of all pertinent patient information. If they could get just this one point from someone who has done the stuff for nearly twenty-five years, great clinical outcomes would soar, and costs would be dramatically reduced; they'd be on par with other developed nations in the world. American medicine is upside down, meaning emphasis has been placed on specialization at the cost of quality and available primary care.

For a doctor to choose primary care and family medicine out of medical school, they need to feel an altruistic call, similar to the ministerial call, due to the low reimbursement, lack of time to spend with patients, burdensome government and health insurance regulations, and extended work hours, which leaves very little personal and family time. So many of our bright medical students would make family medicine their first choice but can't overcome these real and difficult hurdles. They also observe how academia has disrespected primary care and limited their scope of practice so that they become less than what they were trained for.

To reimagine and redesign how family physicians deliver care and how they are reimbursed will take men and women of courage.

They must take their case directly to their patients until others catch up in their thinking. Primary care has been systematically undervalued over a long period of time in the US. The medical-industrial complex has searched for the quick fix while ignoring the real value of primary care and family physicians. These doctors should be the captains of the ship, the navigators of patients' continuous care, and the hub or custodian of their medical records.

Even during the COVID pandemic, the medical-industrial complex watched primary care physicians get further and further behind. Many went out of business due to financial losses during the pandemic. Unfortunately, the system's solution is to reconstruct the payment system into something that is even more complex and convoluted and burdensome, especially to the independent primary care physician. This does not solve the underlying problems. The "leaders" in the medical field seem to feel they need to imagine complex solutions that don't address the core underlying deficits in the practice and profession of primary care. This is like turning up the heat instead of fixing the broken windows. The problem is that many of our "thought leaders" don't do the work and don't see patients day in and day out. They don't know the right questions, much less the answers. One reason for this is their desire for control and power and their unwillingness to consult with independent primary care physicians for solutions.

With this book, I hope to educate patients on membership primary care medicine. Beyond that, I'd like it to be used as a guide for those called to reform health care in the United States to fix primary care, because this is the key to fixing overall health care in our country. If you as a potential healthcare reformer won't make these changes for any other reason, do it to reduce our health care expenses and give us a chance to pay off our enormous financial deficit before Communist China completely owns us and America collapses under its massive debt.

I believe the answer lies in restoring primary care physicians back to their principal role in patient care. Family physicians, who represent the majority of our primary care physicians, are uniquely trained and qualified to manage ninety percent of patients' medical needs in a more efficient and effective manner than the current uncoordinated approach of patients left to see multiple specialists, without any coordination of care from doctor to doctor. Moreover, the primary care physician can coordinate all care with the patient's specialists and hospitals so that the care is better, holistic, and not fragmented—a seamless process for the patient as they move through the healthcare system. Patients are desperate for the family doctor of old, like my former mentor, Dr. C. C. Wannamaker, who worked independently, was patient centered, and provided continuous, coordinated, preventative, and compassionate health care. He was a great example of a family doctor who really knows you and can spend as much time with you as you need. You might say the ideal doctor is a family physician who has Marcus Welby's bedside manner but utilizes modern technology. It's the care patients crave, but this type of family doctor is currently hard to find.

As of 2019, according to *Concierge Medicine Today*, there are only 20,000 of us primary care physicians practicing in this country using a "membership model" of care. Although it represents a small percentage of the roughly one million licensed physicians in the US, membership medicine is growing at a rate of three to six percent annually. However, these numbers are based on interviews, since there is no federal registry or official data base for this information. The membership model of care contracts directly with the patient for services not routinely covered by Medicare or commercial health insurance policies. This approach results in more focus, time, and attention being given to the patient. Instead of taking care of the usual 2,000 to 5,000 patients, the membership doctor is usually taking care of just 200 to 500 patients. The average membership visit is sixty minutes for routine appointments and two hours for new-patient establishing visits and comprehensive physicals.

In contrast, most primary care visits are just seven minutes face to face and fifteen to twenty minutes for annual physicals. In our current system, it's impossible to handle all of a patient's ongoing medical problems. Doctors have to say, "Mrs. Smith, we can only address one problem today at your appointment. If you have other concerns, you will need to schedule another appointment." If Mrs. Smith is at the doctor's office for a follow-up for thyroid labs and a medication refill, but her toes are turning purple, with an oozing ulcer, telling her to schedule another appointment to address the ulcer and its underlying cause is not best care. But either the thyroid or the toe must go unaddressed due to an insufficient time allotment for that visit. The primary care physician, who is trained to treat and manage both problems, will have to refer Mrs. Smith to a specialist because the next patient is waiting, and the doctor is running behind in his or her schedule. Unfortunately, this is the norm with the vast percentage of primary care practices in this country—that is if you can even find a primary care physician in your locale, given the current shortage. Since your primary care doctor can only deal with a single problem in such short amount of time, he or she can only serve as a "feeder" to specialists and hospital systems. This results in expensive, fragmented care, with numerous appointments that the patient must try to navigate on their own. On the other hand, a comprehensive, coordinated, continuous medical care plan can be designed and navigated by the primary care physician, and most of that plan can be addressed in the same office visit. So diagnosis and treatment can be started early, which lowers the likelihood of worsening or complications of a condition.

I'm writing this book during the peak of the COVID-19 pandemic. There is no better example of the misuse of primary care doctors by our society, because this pandemic should have been first dealt with at their level. It was a mistake to put all the pandemic resources into hospital and ICU care. Primary care was again underutilized and undervalued. There's no way to know how much fear could have been dispelled in the population or how many lives may have been saved if the government and the medical-industrial complex would have previously valued and treasured their primary care doctors and encouraged the doctor-patient relationship. Then there would have been a chance to diagnose and treat COVID-19 at the earliest stage of infection, keeping all treatment options available and on the table until new treatments could be discovered and tested.

The Robert Graham Center for Policy Studies in Family Medicine and Primary Care of the American Academy of Family Medicine wrote, "In a given year, roughly 260,000 people are hospitalized for upper respiratory infections. By contrast, 19.5 million patients are seen by primary care physicians for the same condition. One can see from this information that most respiratory infections are not treated at the hospital, but rather at the primary care doctor's office. Since respiratory infection is usually the first manifestation of a COVID infection, why could not the majority of COVID-19 patients have been seen and treated by the primary care physician? Why was there so little emphasis and support of treating COVID at the primary care and community level of care? One can only speculate how many patients may not have been hospitalized or died from COVID if equal resources were made available to the primary care doctors as they were to hospitals, and all treatment options for uncomplicated COVID had been left on the table, including off label use of older existing medications. This is worthy of a serious discussion and debate going forward.

Because primary care has been gutted over the years, the powers to be in medicine (what I term the medical-industrial complex, which is made up of entities such as the federal government and its agencies, for-profit health insurance companies, hospitals, pharmaceutical companies, and the like) essentially took that choice away from the primary care physician and from patients, interfering with the doctor-patient relationship and making potentially effective outpatient treatment for COVID-19 nearly nonexistent. There were a few exceptions; some of our physician heroes went against the medical-industrial complex and treated many patients with practice protocols (protocols based on availability of both past research and on-going clinical experience), such as hydroxychloroquine combined with a Z Pak, or doxycycline and zinc supplementation when there were no other alternatives available at that time—other than supportive care and waiting to see what happens. In other words, the patient gets better, or gets more severely ill requiring hospitalization, ICU admission and even requiring a mechanical ventilator.

This book is intended to educate patients on what to look for and what to request in their primary care physician, and to introduce a small but growing model of care, membership medicine, which has been around for more than two decades but is terribly underutilized; its value and affordability are poorly understood and appreciated. The book also argues that this is a perfect way to supplement care for patients with Medicare insurance (non-HMO), and it works well with private health care insurance PPOs as well.

I hope to demonstrate that the membership model (which some refer to as concierge medicine) is the cornerstone of the transformation of our health care system. It's a model that provides the doctor and patient with the time they need. It focuses on the efficient use of resources to give the patient full use of the doctor's training. It also allows the doctor to fully coordinate all aspects of the patient's health care and wellness journey. In the membership model, patients experience better clinical outcomes and efficient and effective use of health care dollars, with emphasis on wellness and prevention, early detection of disease, and the integration of evidence-based traditional and complementary medicine.

I also present a case for a Christian approach to whole person treatment—body, mind, and spirit. This is what some refer to as a value-based health care proposition, versus a volume-based, assembly-line approach, which has dominated our health care delivery system for many decades due to a fee-for-service payment model that has been terribly unfair to primary care doctors.

Can you imagine how much suffering and death could be avoided and the massive dollars that would be saved if heart attacks and strokes could be prevented. I will be introducing you to the BaleDoneen Method later in the book that deals with this very topic. This method prevents these common but horrible and catastrophic cardiovascular events. Many membership practices are practicing this method, or one similar, in cardiovascular care.

Membership medicine allows the patient to age more gracefully and with less chronic disease and disability. Patients give the relationship with their membership family physicians the highest marks for satisfaction; therefore, the doctors practicing in this model retain over ninety-seven percent of the patients from year to year. Since membership primary care was started the mid-1990s, this approach has been shown, over and over, to significantly reduce emergency room visits and hospitalizations, and, therefore, costs.

Come with me on this journey of defining all the wonderful benefits of membership medicine. I predict you will have a paradigm shift in your thinking and desire this kind of relationship that your parents and grandparents had with their family physician, who really knew them as patients and friends. They experienced an unhurried exam and excellence of care. You can have this with the added benefit of modern technology for the cost of a gourmet cup of coffee daily. That seems a small price to pay for superior health care. Make your health your first expense, not your last. For just the amount of a modest utility bill, you can move from a fragmented, disjointed, and often a broken and frustrating health care experience to one that guides you through all the twists and turns in a seamless and efficient manner. Imagine having your personal physician no further away than a text or phone call, who can integrate with your health insurance to give you the best of both worlds. Your health insurance is not health care. What are you waiting for? Let's get started on your new and exciting health care journey. If you decide to join with a membership primary care physician, you'll never regret your decision. It will likely save or prolong your life and prevent unforeseen health care costs from causing your personal bankruptcy. "An ounce of prevention is worth a pound of cure."

Chapter 1

DEMAND FOR FAMILY PHYSICIANS IS GREAT, BUT NOT WITHOUT CHALLENGES

What would you attempt to do if you knew you could not fail?
—Unknown

For with God nothing shall be impossible.
—Luke 1:37 (KJV)

Many specialists in medicine call themselves primary care doctors, but I want to make the argument that the only true primary care doctor is the family physician. With their broad scope of practice and training, they can serve as your primary care specialist. Family physicians are unique in that they are the only specialty of medicine that treats the whole person, taking into consideration their patients' biopsychosocial and family dynamics and their values. They are trained to treat the whole family, from the womb to the tomb. Certainly, we have some general internists who serve as adult primary care doctors, but their numbers have severely shrunk in recent decades; over two thirds of general internists elect to continue on in training to become a medical specialist which are numerous, such as cardiology, gastroenterology, and pulmonology, just to mention a few. A medical or surgical specialist differs from a primary care doctor in that their scope or field of practice is severely narrowed into a single organ system such as heart, lungs, gastrointestinal tract, etc. With only one third of general internists serving as adult primary care doctors, their numbers have been further reduced in the outpatient-practice setting with many of these choosing to function as full-time hospitalists, with ninety percent of our hospitalists being general internists and only ten percent family physicians. Then of course we have pediatricians, who are primary care doctors for our babies and younger children, and OB/GYN doctors have a limited primary care role in women's health as they're in a surgical specialty. OB/GYN doctors are limited and more specialized in their scope of medical expertise. For example, since heart attacks are the most common cause of death in post-menopausal women, not breast cancer, women are typically better served by having a family physician or general internist handle most, if not all of, their medical care, even if they choose to get their gynecologic services from a GYN specialist.

Family physicians are by far the most heavily recruited physicians in the country and make up the highest percentage of physician shortages in the US. Unfortunately, the heavy workload, paperwork, regulations, overhead to run their practices, and the lowest Medicare and commercial health care insurance reimbursements of any physician groups, this has caused thousands to leave their profession for a career outside patient care or take early retirement. This adversarial environment and lack of prestige in the medical community discourages many of our medical students from pursuing careers in family medicine, even though it is by far the most attractive to many of our medical students, especially to our older and more experienced students. This is because it's comprehensive and crosses over into all the medical specialties. It's the only medical specialty that is "whole person medicine," since it treats the whole person, body, mind, and spirit, and relating each single organ system to all of the other organ systems in the body. It has been the primary care physicians who have typically been the physician specialists to integrate alternative and complementary medicine into their practice as well.

There is broad recognition of the central role of primary care in the nation's health care–delivery system. Up until around 2008, health workforce projections largely neglected primary care. Baseline projections produce a greater shortage in primary care than in any other specialty area of medicine. Projections suggest that by 2025, more than a third of the overall physician shortage will be in primary care, or about 46,000 full time primary care physicians. As of the writing of this book, we are less than five years away from this staggering number. This was made worse by the permanent loss of independent primary care physicians during the COVID-19 crisis, when many were not able to survive the economic shutdown, the orders to shelter at home, and their own patients' fear of going into to the doctor's office, where they felt they might be more exposed to the virus. Also, the older population in the US is growing rapidly, while the growth of the younger population has been much slower. And the younger generation is having fewer children and more abortions (over sixty-two million since 1973).

Even worse, many students are talked out of going into family medicine by their medical school professors and faculty because these older doctors view family medicine as inferior and subservient to medical specialists. To fully appreciate this, we only need to look back to a time prior to World War II, when most of our physicians were family doctors or generalists, with general internists serving as specialists for hospitalized patients and the general surgeon. In many cities and towns, the family doctor handled all the obstetrics and many common and routine general surgeries, such as appendectomy and hernia repairs.

After World War II, the United States had an explosion of specialization training and fellowships in medicine and surgery, and little by little, the scope of practice for the family physician and the general surgeon began to be whittled away by our specialists in the medical and surgical fields. The public was told through media that medicine was improved by seeing a "specialist," which was always superior to seeing a "generalist." Our specialists believed this with all their might. They taught medical school students the same, and they demanded and fought for better reimbursement, creating associations and political action committees (PACs) to fight for them in Washington, DC, which has continued until today.

With the advent of third-party medical payments in the 1960s—with the passage of Medicare and Medicaid—specialist societies fought like honey baggers for better and better government and commercial health insurance reimbursement, tying it to procedures more than to cognitive skills and patient education. Family medicine didn't even get into the game of having a PAC to fight for their members for fair reimbursement until the 2000s, at which time the financial resources had been heavily leveraged in Medicare and Medicaid. Too little too late, you might say.

The large commercial health insurance companies saw an opportunity to control and even limit their reimbursement to primary care physicians. They accomplished this by tying their reimbursements to primary physicians as a percentage of Medicare allowable reimbursement. Thus, they did not pay the primary care physician their full professional rate and for that matter neither did Medicare. This is one method employed by for profit health insurance companies to help generate larger profits for their shareholders and high salaries and bonuses for their CEOs and other senior employees. Even more problematic was that the American

Medical Association (AMA) created the relative value update committee (RUC) to determine, on a yearly basis, the Medicare physician reimbursement schedule, which highly favored procedures performed by specialists and paid for the supplies and facility costs for their procedures and visits. They then paid primary care physicians less for the same work. For example, if a dermatologist removes a suspicious mole, they're paid at a higher rate than a primary care physician. Also, the dermatologist gets paid for a "surgical kit," which would include the supplies used for the surgery, whereas the supplies used by a primary care physician would be bundled, and he or she would only be paid for the overall surgery and would have to eat the cost of supplies. As a caring physician, I have patients who expect that I will bandage their wounds, which is a real cost to me as a solo primary care physician, but Medicare and commercial health insurances will only pay if the wound is a burn, not any other kind of common wound. The severely discounted payments to family physicians, even for noncovered or bundled services and supplies, are a concept that patients don't really understand. With the high insurance rates, they pay and the high out-of-pocket copays and deductibles, they can't fathom the idea that their doctor is not being fairly reimbursed.

Before the 1992 implementation of the Medicare fee schedule, physician payments were made under the "usual, customary, and reasonable" payment model (a charge-based payment system). Physician services were largely considered to be mis-valued under this system, with evaluation and management services being undervalued and procedures overvalued. Third-party payers (public and private health insurance) advocated an improved model to replace the usual, customary, and reasonable (UCR) fees, which had been associated with stark examples of specialists making significantly higher sums of money from third party payers than primary care physicians. These payments to specialists could amount to tens of millions of dollars more over the course of a career than their primary care physician colleagues.

Primary care physicians were hopeful every time changes were made to health care, because these changes would mean a better reimbursement for them for the cognitive work that goes into diagnosing every organ system in the body; educating the patient; and diagnosing, treating, managing, and preventing chronic disease. But so far, the changes have not translated into enough reimbursement for students to be incentivized into choosing primary care as a specialty. Also, family physicians' own association bought into the lie that primary care physicians had to document and electronically prove that what they were already doing was valuable so they could be paid a little more. They worked with health insurances, the AMA, and with the government to burden primary care physicians with "proofs of work" requirements, and encouragement to join accountable care organizations (ACO) to gain another 5 percent in reimbursement. What many physicians didn't realize was that shortly after signing up for the ACO, they would begin to be fined or have their payments reduced if they didn't meet the requirements to save dollars in the care of these patients. For ACO physicians to be paid a little more, they're required to share in the risk of financial losses with the commercial health insurance company.

So let's compare the work of the specialist to the comprehensiveness of the primary care physician. This is not to say that specialists deal with less complexity, but I would argue that few of them deal with more, because their field of work is limited to one organ system. Primary care doctors must know an enormous amount of detail about all organ systems, how they function, symptoms of medical problems within that system, the tests that would provide a definitive diagnosis, and what procedures or treatments would be needed to mitigate or manage the disease. An integrated membership family physician even goes a step further in identifying the root causes of diseases with earlier detection, reversal, and prevention of the disease condition.

I have had a long medical career, spanning more than five decades, including an academic career in clinical pharmacy and pharmacology, scientific surgical research and administration, teaching in medical schools at Mayo Clinic and Creighton University Schools of Medicine and Pharmacy, and nearly twenty-five years in private practice in family medicine. I likely would not have gone into family medicine had I not done externships outside the medical center and observed some outstanding family physicians practicing in the community in urban, suburban, and rural areas of the Midwest. What I discovered in working with these outstanding family physicians that impressed me so was how they functioned minute by minute, day in and day out, across all the specialty areas of medicine and outpatient surgical procedures, diagnosing and treating so many different disease states in a whole-person, comprehensive, patient-centered way. When I rotated through the offices of specialists in medicine and surgery as a medical student, I was impressed with how these specialists had advanced the science in their respective areas but practiced like "partialists," generally dealing with just one organ system.

I noticed an interesting trend; more than 50 percent of the patients they saw in their offices—either new patients or those following up—were easily handled by a family physician, if only we had enough time and if there were enough of us. Over the years, we had many of our older workhorse family physicians leave our great specialty due to the frustration of regulations forced upon them by the federal government and lack of reimbursement. As a result, specialists became overwhelmed with primary care patients and had to hire nurse practitioners and physician assistants to handle their heavy office work loads. It was not that many years ago that family physicians and general internists saw two thirds of all outpatient visits. Patients are being scheduled for multiple visits to specialists' offices for multiple follow-up visits that could be managed by the primary care physician. If the patients were established with a membership physician, their doctor could easily manage the ongoing, stable medical problems the patient may have. Sometimes a patient would present to a specialist's office for the initial visit and were not seen by the doctor but rather the nurse practitioner or physician assistant at all follow-up visits. Don't get me wrong; many of our advanced clinicians are outstanding health care professionals and individuals. I welcome them into the medical field and there is plenty of room for their unique contributions, but we should not be cranking them out in record numbers, because our system is completely broken and depleted of primary care physicians.

Primary care means first care—foundational care. Strong health care starts with strong primary care, and until our health care system is fixed properly, we will continue to have a broken, dysfunctional, disjointed health care–delivery system in the United States that too often is driven by greed, power, control, and the wrong motives in our stake holders, where physicians and patients don't have a seat at the table. Fix primary care and family medicine, and you reform health care in general for the better. And you save an incredible amount of money that could go a long way toward paying off our ever-growing $28 trillion national debt and fund Medicare for years to come. This national debt exploded in 2020, due to several federal stimulus bills passed by Congress because of the economic devastation of lockdowns of entire industries in attempt to limit the spread of COVID infections, only to see it peak again when the lockdowns are lifted. As President Trump said, "The treatment cannot be worse than the disease." Now it is the Democrats turn to run all the federal government, and they have a history of increased deficit spending, so our financial plight will likely worsen. Even more reason to fix primary care.

For example, if a patient has uncontrolled diabetes for decades, and they must have their leg amputated, the costs to the insurance payer for the surgeon and hospital for that procedure are tremendous. If that same patient is in a membership medicine practice, with comprehensive prevention and diabetic education, labs every three months, and dietary and exercise counseling, the leg, foot, and toes would be potentially saved, the patient would not go onto dialysis and would probably never have a heart attack. Such a patient can live a long, productive life. Which course is more expensive? To the patient, which is more valuable? Why has this not been pointed out? Who's benefiting the most by not making the changes? Health insurance companies don't have the incentives to pay more for prevention because most of the sickest are Medicare age, and they're paid for by the government. A government doesn't change unless it's forced to by the public and by strong decisive leadership in medicine. This must be practical, righteous, and wise. Unfortunately these qualities are severely lacking in those who hold power in government and academia and professional societies. I believe the hunger for greed and power has corrupted much of our leadership and has influenced medical policies. Unfortunately, practicing physicians have little influence in health care delivery and policy. This is particularly sad, because it's the doctors providing the care who will know what's best for their patients and the country, not bureaucrats.

The bottom line is that medicine desperately needs more family physicians functioning at the top of their scope of practice in the United States, and they need to be paid for the work that they do. The problem, unfortunately, goes far beyond not having enough. They need more time—much more time—and fewer patients on their panels to take care of properly. They need more resources to do their jobs effectively. And they need to be supported and respected as equals by our specialty colleagues, the medical-industrial complex, and even by our own academy and peers. Our Academy of Family Physicians should be censured for saying that family physicians are not fully adequate and functional. Such doctors should not have to keep jumping through more performance hoops to gain the respect and support they deserve. This is a betrayal of our specialty and its members. Never again should a family physician believe or be told that a specialist is superior, even though the former are paid less by third-party payers for the exact same work. This must be fixed, even if it means lengthening our family medicine residency training from three years to a total of four or five years.

We don't have the time or patience to hope, pray, and wish that the medical-industrial complex will change in my lifetime. I would be better off in my work and reimbursement if I practiced in England, Australia, or anywhere but the good ol' USA. In those other countries, I could enjoy the full scope of my practice and receive fair and competitive reimbursements. I'd also have a level of professional independence, with prevention as the focus. But the US is my country. I love this country and its citizens, and I have personally experienced a better and more perfect primary care model, both as a membership primary care physician and as one who pays his own personal physician, who also has a membership practice. In other words, I have personally experienced the tremendous value of membership medicine as both a doctor and as a patient.

I'm proposing a proven model of membership primary care that allows family physicians or general internists to practice independently, so they can put the patient and only the patient first and give them the time and resources and integrated services that will make their care extremely valuable. If adopted widely in our country, it will result in much better outcomes, save our patients a lot of pain and suffering, and save our health care system a tremendous amount of money. We can't continue to pay twice as much for our health care as the next country in the developed world and have much worse health outcomes than so many other countries; the US is ranked thirty-seventh in the world in overall health.

The answer is not socialism and regulation; it simply won't work in the United States and is *not* compatible with our constitution and bill of rights, which grants its citizens inalienable rights, not government control over our lives. The answer is innovative reform of primary care, allowing the patient to have real health care, not just health insurance and end-stage disease care. This innovative model of membership primary care should be universally attractive to employed patients, specialists, hospitals, the government, health insurance companies, and especially to primary care physicians. Health insurance companies need to get out of the business of practicing and regulating medicine. This is a conflict of interest and makes them beholden to shareholders more than to the patients who are paying their premiums. For our needy, we need to pool our governmental and charitable resources to fix and grow excellent community health centers, like the effective reforms in the Veterans Administration (VA) system under the Trump administration, but with the addition of faith-based charitable programs. The membership model may not work for all of our population, but it's already quietly growing at a rate of six percent annually. At this rate, its ranks will grow rapidly and to a much larger number than the current 20,000 membership doctors in the US.

Chapter 2

WHY IS IT VITAL TO HAVE AN INDEPENDENT MEMBERSHIP FAMILY PHYSICIAN?

The practice of medicine is an art, not a trade; a calling, not a business; a calling in which your heart will be exercised equally with your head. Often the best part of your work will have nothing to do with potions and powders, but with the exercise of an influence of the strong upon the weak, of the righteous upon the wicked, of the wise upon the foolish.
—Sir William Osler (1849–1919)

It is difficult to get a man to understand something when his salary depends upon his not understanding it.
—Upton Sinclair

Every modernized country in the world, other than the United States, understands that without a primary care foundation, you don't have a successful health care–delivery system. Why has this been such a problem in the US? First, with the specialization of medicine after World War II, the general practitioner was gradually becoming more and more inferior in the minds of academia and medical societies, which emphasized surgical centers as those centers became more and more prominent in their hearts and minds with breakthroughs in medical discoveries, surgeries, and emergency medicine. Primary care physicians were moving from the cornerstone of health care delivery to the position of a cold-and-cough doctor and a triage and referral agent for specialists and hospital services.

Also, specialists wanted the family physician to become the "scut monkey" (a term used for medical students who perform the busy undesirable work for their supervising physicians in patient care; an inferior physician) for them in the overall health care of patients in the hospital and outpatient clinics. In other words, specialists were touted as having superior expertise in diagnosing and treating all medical problems, while it was the job of the family doctor to handle routine, self-limiting health issues, such as coughs and colds, and to determine which medical specialist to refer the patient to. The specialist would take over the care and, in many cases, have the patient return to them regularly for chronic disease management. A family physician was looked upon by many in the medical-industrial complex as inferior to specialists in making an accurate diagnosis, as well as managing patients' ongoing chronic diseases. The primary care doctor was watching his or her scope of practice (i.e., what they can diagnose, treat, and manage) diminish as specialists gained more respect and influence in the medical field.

In reality, in other advanced countries, the family doctor is the hub of health care, representing 50 percent or more of all doctors in those countries, and has a broad scope of practice. Only the sickest and most challenging patients and those with complex disease states (for which the primary care physician requires help) are referred to specialists, because, as pointed out in the introduction, the primary care physician can manage ninety percent of the problems presented on a day-to-day basis.

There is a host of reasons why the primary care physician is vital to optimizing health care in a community, and the transformation of family medicine is essential to successful health care reform in the United States. The late Dr. Barbara Starfield, Director of Primary Care Study and Research at Johns Hopkins School of Medicine, wrote:

> When studied from county to county across the United States when a community was over penetrated with specialists and short on primary care physicians, health outcomes were worse, and costs were much higher. The converse was true, the more highly penetrated a county was with primary care physicians and less so with specialists, the better were health outcomes of the citizens and the costs were much lower. "Studies in the early 1990s showed that those U.S. states with higher ratios of primary care physicians to population had better health outcomes, including lower rates of all causes of mortality: mortality from heart disease, cancer, or stroke; infant mortality; low birth weight; and poor self-reported health, even after controlling for sociodemographic measures (percentages of elderly, urban, and minority; education; income; unemployment; pollution) and lifestyle factors (seatbelt use, obesity, and smoking) subsequently showed that the supply of primary care physicians was associated with an increase in life span and with reduced low birth-weight rates." Starfield, B., S. Leiyu, and J. Macinko. "Primary Care Contribution to Health Systems and Health." *Milbank Q 83(8) 2005:457-502.*

This has not been widely discussed in medicine and among those entities that make up the medical-industrial complex because it runs counter to the notion—popular for the past seventy-five years—that specialists are superior because of their advanced training, with rescue medicine being prioritized instead of prevention. It always makes me chuckle how some specialists hold the primary care physician to their standard in their more narrow field, yet could they manage so many areas of medicine (from A to Z) as effectively if they had the job of a primary care doctor?

In this situation, rather than have one doctor, the family physician, coordinate specialty care, specialists routinely refer patients to other specialists. This results in what might be called "polymedicine." In other words, patients can end up with too many doctors taking care of them, resulting in uncoordinated, fragmented medical care with no one physician seeing the whole medical picture of that patient. You might be surprised to learn that the average Medicare patient has up to twelve specialists handling their medical care. And unless the patient is fortunate enough to have a membership primary care physician to oversee and coordinate their care among many specialists, the patient is typically on their own, without primary care navigation and care coordination.

In a smaller, membership-based practice (200 to 500 patients total) the membership primary care physician and team is tracking every test ordered and every specialist's office note or procedure. He or she reads every word of the results and doctors notes and makes sure everything the specialist has recommended is followed up on and completed. They do this to make sure those recommendations don't conflict with the other medical problems the patient has or the medications or supplements they're taking. Unfortunately, specialists often refer to other specialists, rather than communicating with the primary care physician.

Those specialist-to-specialist referrals require extra work and coordination to get those office notes and test results back to the primary care physician. It introduces one or more specialists, possibly outside the referral network of the primary care physician. Sometimes, we feel like a cat chasing its tail. While the original specialist may have meant for this to be useful, it only creates more work and the potential for uncoordinated and fragmented patient care when the referrals flow from specialist to specialist to specialist. This drives up health care costs and often can lead to poor patient compliance and poor outcomes. Patients desire to have one physician they can go to for help with understanding their options and the risks and benefits of procedures. They want a doctor who speaks their language and will serve as their advocate in an often uncoordinated and fragmented health care system that can seem very impersonal at times. Even poor follow-up and communication by the doctor's staff leaves them feeling insecure, and they begin to lose trust and confidence in the specialist, who may be excellent, but doesn't have the time or interest to personally lead his team and hold them accountable for excellent patient care and communication with the patient's primary care physician.

It's unfortunate that the original specialists don't appreciate the intense role we perform in a membership relationship with the patient, but since it's so rare for the primary care physician to provide these services these days—when time is so limited with the patient—I can understand why it happens. Family physicians should have the time and resources to reduce their patient panel size to one that's manageable—under five hundred patients, not two to five thousand. They should routinely provide oversight services and ongoing care coordination among all physicians taking care of the patient.

In conversation with individuals asking about my practice, I can't tell you how many times their second or third question is how many patients I have in my practice. The implication is that the larger the number, the more successful I am as a doctor. Some primary care doctors proudly announce how many thousands of patients they're taking care of, even inflating that number, when in fact, they've only seen half the numbers they state in the last two years. Many are simply lost to follow-up because the primary care doctor and his or her staff are too busy and overwhelmed to even check on them. I would suggest that's not something we as family physicians should be proud of or even accept. It reflects how little time, devotion, and quality medical care these thousands of patients are actually receiving. If we're working in a system that's not functioning properly, how can we be the patient's advocate? We simply need time and the resources to function as the patient navigator, and having too many patients adds to our problem of lack of both time and resources. And I would contend this contributes to poorer patient outcomes and physician burn-out.

The patient needs an independent advocate who's not beholden to their health insurance or the health care system. They need someone who can fight for them or have the alternatives available when the system is so broken that patients can't work through the maze of complexity to get the care they need. Is solo practice the answer for primary care? One commentator noted an amazingly simple solution, though it runs counter to current employment trends among physicians. His answer to non-medical persons deciding what's best for the medical professionals was to go out on his own. He points out that it may not be economically feasible for many, but for him it was just too bitter a pill to swallow having people who only give a hoot about the bottom line dictating to him how to do his job, telling him he had to see more patients faster and faster, on top of meeting after meeting stealing his precious time. Another physician, who was terminated from his hospital position for speaking out about patient care, said he felt fortunate in solo practice after enduring the abuses of the hospital system. He went on to point out that he always thought it perverse that hospitals gave out privileges and charged primary care doctors hundreds of dollars per year to come to their facility. It's the doctors who are doing all the work, bring in the patients to the hospital facility and enduring the liability. He said, "When will physicians wake up?"

If we can't push back against the pressure to be less than what we were trained to be, then the primary care doctor becomes a piece-rate worker, focused on, and forced to see large volumes of patients every day, as fast as possible, to make a living. Unfortunately, it's a vicious cycle, because as the number of patients increases, more and more support staff and supplies are needed. Overhead skyrockets, forcing most to go to work for large hospital systems to pay for school loans and support growing families.

Primary care doctors think they've solved their overhead burden by being employed, but they haven't gotten off the treadmill and are now working for "the system," not necessarily the patient. At that point, it becomes illness triage and rescue care, not the gold standard of prevention, early detection of disease, and lifestyle counseling that's critical for a patient's long-term health. With such an approach, health care becomes more cost efficient, less dysfunctional, more proactive, and more coordinated. Preventing and reversing diabetes mellitus, heart attacks, stroke, and cancer radically transforms how we delivery health care in the US and cuts our costs to a fraction of what we're currently paying. Deregulating health care will further improve it at all levels and inspire doctors to stay in the profession and enjoy their work again.

All the above is why the primary care physician needs to be independent, and the only model that makes this possible currently is membership primary care. I will talk more about how we got to such a dysfunctional and abusive place in the chapter on how health insurance is not health care. This has resulted in a crisis in our health care system, which has been brought to light with the COVID pandemic. We have weak and ineffective community health, severely depleted primary care, and a lack of adequate reimbursement to support a primary care doctor's time with patients. This is the great health care crisis of our time.

Independent primary care physicians have no ability to negotiate their contracts with Medicare, Medicaid, or commercial insurance companies, unlike the local hospital system or large numbers of specialists billing under one insurance number. Independent primary care doctors can take it or leave it regarding health insurance contracts, but to accept their payment means that, under the insurance-based reimbursement system and Medicare (thanks to the AMA and their RUC), we are paid about forty to fifty cents on the dollar, and commercial insurance companies often get away with paying even less than Medicare to primary care physicians. Still, they pay specialists in full. This is ethically and morally wrong. The Bible states that a worker is worth his wages (Matt. 10:10, Luke 10:7, I Tim. 5:18).

Contrast this with a hospital-employed primary care doctor receiving eighty to one hundred percent more in reimbursement than those in independent practice. Subspecialist receive up to 300 percent above Medicare from commercial plans. No wonder those specialists that are popular and busy can afford to drop Medicare patients, which contributes to the ever-growing shortage for our oldest and neediest patients.

The problem is that independent family physicians with large, insurance-based practices are feeders to the hospitals and specialists. These patients, who are referred to specialists by family physicians, bring to the hospital and those specialties the most dollars of all referral sources, often exceeding one million dollars annually per health care system per family physician. Rarely does the hospital or specialist refer patients to a primary care physician. You would think that since we were the number one economic referral source, there would be appreciation and respect, but in return, the hospital charges outpatient primary care physicians annual dues of hundreds of dollars just to be able to provide documentation for third party payers, Medicare, and commercial insurances. They're required to be on a hospital staff to participate in health care plans. Contrast this to the subspecialists, who are supported by the hospital with expensive surgical equipment, surgical suites, surgical staff, and medical specialists, who do procedures to support their work. Proceduralists provide more direct hospital income, whereas primary care doctors bring more indirect income via referrals. What responsibility does the local hospital bear regarding the demise of primary care in their communities?

The latest reports indicate that over 50 percent of *all* doctors are now employed, mainly by hospitals. The pressure of seeing too many patients in a day does not go away when primary physicians are employed. The employing hospitals will sometimes play games to see how many patients the primary care physician can see in one hour. Those moving the quickest through the large numbers of patients are given verbal accolades, rewards, prizes, and bonuses to shame those that might wish to give their patients the most valuable commodity they possess, their time. It is well known that employed female primary care physicians make annual incomes less than their male counterpart. One reason for this was recently brought to light. Women physicians will spend 2.6 more minutes per visit with their patients, and this adds up to a significantly lower number of patients they're able to see annually, and this results in lower income.

So, when family physicians give up their practice and independence, they solve their inability to cover their overhead and expenses but relinquish their independence to their new employer, the hospital system. This can be literally deadly for their patients, and it's all in the name of the employer or hospital trying to make the family doctors cover their salary, benefits, and some of the hospital overhead. The hospitals often fail to appreciate how much value and indirect financial benefit one employed family physician brings to their institutions. They totally miss the fact that the ultimate quality of patient care, patient satisfaction, and clinical outcomes rests more at the primary care level than the specialty level of care.

Family medicine doctors are the Cinderellas of medicine. They're much like the Israelites in the Bible when they were in slavery in Egypt and were forced to make bricks without straw (Exod. 5:7). Great primary care can only happen when the doctor and the patient have adequate time together face to face. The primary care doctor must have a generous amount of time to coordinate care of the patient as he or she moves through the often disorganized and dysfunctional aspects of outpatient and inpatient treatment and testing. One of the ongoing gross dysfunctions around the country is in the process of discharging a patient from the hospital and getting them back into the care of the primary care physician. When this is not performed well, not only can medication errors and patient noncompliance occur, but more frequent rehospitalizations can occur to the hospital and adversely affect their quality-of-care scores. Most recently, I even had an experience in which a hospitalist "stole" my patient after he took care of him during a hospitalization for pneumonia. The patient didn't know any better. He was just being compliant with the instructions of the hospitalist instead of me, his primary care doctor. Of course, this is absolutely against hospital policy and is unethical behavior on the part of the hospitalist.

Years ago, I suggested to our local hospital leadership team that they take some of their profits (technically they are a nonprofit hospital, and hospitals are generally very profitable) and invest it in a center of excellence for primary care, in our Scottsdale community. This would be run by and benefit both the independent and employed primary care physicians. Rather than doing that, our local hospital system just announced the purchase of the majority share of a popular ambulatory urgent care center company with centers across all of Arizona. These urgent care facilities, both free standing and in drug store chains, compete with our primary care physicians. In other words, they take the "easy" acute visits and leave the primary care doctor with the most difficult chronic disease management and care coordination, which they only have seven minutes per visit to deal with.

I would like to share a story of how an urgent care facility can distract from patients getting that quality comprehensive continuous primary care. My sister Mary was diagnosed with colon cancer. She underwent extensive surgery, radiation, and six months of chemotherapy when she was in her forties. Her best friend was with her through all this. You would think she'd have taken her cue from Mary's situation and gotten established with a primary care physician who would do regular colon screenings for cancer. Instead, she used an urgent care physician as her primary care doctor, only seeing him for acute medical problems as they occurred. When the patient reached the age of sixty, she had never had a colon cancer screening. Quite likely, it had never even been suggested to her. She found herself with breathing problems that eventually landed her into the hospital. She was found to have out-of-control blood sugars, and after proceeding with a workup, she was found to have metastatic colon cancer. From my point of view, her suffering and death were needless. If only she'd had a regular primary care physician who emphasized prevention, likely she would have been screened regularly for colon cancer. Ironically, her metastatic colon cancer was only discovered after hospital discharge when she became established with a primary care physician. Unfortunately, she suffered prolonged chemotherapy and an agonizing death. This was so sad and tragic, and it emphasizes the fact that urgent care can't assume the role of primary care.

Dr. Starfield was not a family physician but a pediatrician, and she recognized that there was something unique and inherently valuable in the way family doctors interacted with their patients that was not at all similar to any other medical specialty. This uniqueness is described as treating the patients' wholistic health. The family physician sees the patient's ability to function within their biopsychosocial environment—with their family and friends, on the job, and within their spheres of influence in their world and community. This is more important than treating an organ system in the body and fitting a diagnosis into a tightly packaged and wrapped box we call a medical diagnosis.

Unfortunately, we as physicians are forced to categorize diagnoses by dealing with an alphanumeric system of fitting the patient into a coding system called ICD-10, which contains more than 60,000 different diagnostic disease codes. And family doctors have to code more broadly than any other medical specialists. If this were not enough to drive your physician crazy, our required billing system for various aspects of the patients' care is complex. It relies on the use of CPT codes, and if a doctor gets them wrong, he or she can be charged with fraud. Can you imagine the burden it might place on your accountant or attorney if they had to bill you for their services in this manner? They simply bill for their time at a specific rate, and so should physicians.

You might believe it couldn't get any worse, but there's also documentation required for quality assurance measurements. Physicians must document what they did for the patient and what the medical-industrial complex has determined is quality and is not. The most complicated documentation is called MIPS. As stated before, our own academy has bought the lie, told over the last seventy-five years by the medical-industrial complex, that family doctors are inferior to specialists and are not uniquely qualified after education and training. So how do we as family physicians convince anyone in the medical community that many of us chose the family medicine specialty not because we had to, but because we thought it was special and possibly one of the most challenging specialties when performed to our full potential?

All this bureaucracy and wasted time and effort on things that have nothing to do with great patient care are a recipe for physician burn out. We're thought of as second-class physicians because we are "only" family physicians. We're taken advantage of as "scut monkeys," (see previous definition) paid impossibly low and immoral reimbursements by government and third-party payers, not allowed to have the time to practice or utilize our expertise, and forced to deal with a narrowed scope of practice. This is why many family physicians are leaving patient care, which is what attracted them to medicine in the first place. Or they're simply being pushed out of practice into a new career or early retirement. If I've heard it once, I've heard it a thousand times. When ask, "Well what kind of doctor are you?" some primary care doctors say, "Oh, just a general practitioner." This is wrong. We should say, "A whole-person specialist and the patient's primary doctor."

It's like the story of the ugly sisters and Cinderella, the fairest of them all, who was left at home to clean the house while the selfish sisters went to the party. Not taking anything away from our specialists, but truth be known, so many of our brightest and best medical students would prefer to specialize in family medicine if it paid better, if there was more respect for the specialty, and if the work were better supported with the resources that would allow us to treat fewer patients with more time and caring and thoroughness.

The obvious key to health care reform is foundational, implementing the first principals of good health care, and that is providing good patient primary care. An independent primary care physician providing personalized primary care is the answer, but these heroes of medicine must get out of a volume reimbursement and enter a deregulated environment of practice. They must be given the time and resources and the reasonable patient load that will allow them to help patients maneuver through a dysfunctional and fragmented health care system. In addition, malpractice reform is needed in states where there is no cap on damages for pain and suffering. Only when this happens will we see patient satisfaction and health outcomes truly blossom.

A well-known practice model, membership medicine, has had over two decades to work out the kinks and is ready to be looked at seriously as one of the best models for returning family physicians to their place of importance and centrality in patient care, with full functionality and respect. Our patients will benefit, the health care system will benefit, and the high cost of fragmented health care in the US will drop dramatically. Only imagine if heart attacks, strokes, diabetes, and some cancers could be prevented by early detection and intervention, focusing on the root causes that drive the disease. Guess what; they can be, but it takes time, resources, and willingness of the doctor to reject the status quo and adopt new concepts (such as the Bale Doneen heart attack and stroke prevention that will be discussed in a later chapter). It will take some convincing of patients and the medical-industrial complex, but when the patient demands this model, nothing can stop it. It is like any new idea; it's first rejected, then ostracized, then accepted, and finally celebrated. Membership primary care physicians have been pioneers since the mid-1990s, and after twenty-five years of success, membership primary care is ready to be celebrated. Are we getting closer to a tipping point in the transformation for the specialty of family medicine? The current scarcity of primary care doctors, and certainly their lack of time for the patient, is driving a desire and need for membership primary care.

Chapter 3

How to Identify a Family Physician who Is Personal, Compassionate, and Scientific

It has always seemed a strange paradox to me that the man in medicine who needs the greatest knowledge of all has the shortest period of training, and the man who needs knowledge in a very narrow segment of medicine or surgery has years of training before he enters practice. It has been my observation that the general practitioner is often the real doctor and the specialist is often a superior mechanic in a narrow field.
—William Standish Reed, MD

Data should act as the foundation for your decision-making process, not as a substitute for your own judgement. Different tools and techniques are required with the individual patient.
—Phillip O. Katz, MD

In the world of membership primary care, a patient should be looking for a physician who's caring, personal, compassionate, and willing to give the time necessary to develop a personal, trusting relationship with the patient. That way, a therapeutic alliance can develop, and effective medical transactions can be carried out. I like to refer to this as a process in which the doctor and the patient labor together for the improvement of the patient's health and well-being. Years ago, this was the case with patients and their primary doctors or family physicians, until the medical-industrial complex got involved and started telling physicians what to do. This was a direct interference with the doctor-patient relationship, and it reduced the amount of quality time a doctor could spend with a patient by placing all sorts of regulatory and documentation demands on the physician.

Spending time with patients is critical for prevention and early detection of disease. Unfortunately, today, most primary care doctors are limited to only seven minutes of face-to-face time with the patient, and because they need to fill up their schedules with many appointments, they must see twenty-five to forty patients a day. So a family doctor must have a panel of patients ranging from 2,000 to 5,000 to fill up the schedule every day. Until COVID, the only way most primary care doctors got paid was to see the patient directly in the office. Just recently, a telemedicine visit began to be paid at a rate similar to (but still less than) that of an in-person visit, but this reimbursement policy was approved only through the duration of COVID pandemic. Congress will now have to be willing to implement President Trump's call to make telemedicine reimbursements equal to in-office visits permanently.

Can you see how reimbursement based solely on face-to-face office visits simply does not work in favor of the patient. Usually only one medical problem can be addressed per visit, and even so, the doctor may not have enough time to deal with a more complex problem. With only seven minutes to deal with a patient face to face, often there simply isn't enough time for the family doctor to work out what the problem is, and it gets quickly referred to the specialist. Referral to a specialist takes less time than to work it up and manage the medical issue. The primary care doctor then serves as a "feeder" to the specialist. With so many patients to take care of, the primary care doctor often doesn't even know your name until he or she looks at the chart before entering the room. Often the therapeutic alliance never gets past the acquaintance stage, so trusted medical transactions can't possibly take place. Because of lack of education and buy-in by the patient, the patient may be noncompliant with recommended therapies. Even worse, the patient may not follow up with the doctor because they've experienced a sub-par medical visit in which too little time was spent, and a therapeutic alliance was simply not formed.

What most patients and family physicians want is sufficient time to handle the patient's needs, complaints of symptoms, or questions regarding chronic disease management. The doctor may also need to address serious acute problems the patient may also present with. Education of the patient results in better compliance and by-in by the patient, but this one activity takes the most time, and if it occurs at all, it's often delegated to an allied health professional of lesser education and training. Of course, it takes more income to employ ancillary health care professionals, and this means seeing more patients daily, which again hinders the doctor-patient relationship due to insufficient doctor-patient time together.

You can see how this is a vicious cycle. The doctor has to go faster and faster and has less and less time with the most important person in the office—*the patient*. In the current primary care practice model, there is less time for early detection of disease and reversal, wellness strategies, and unique programs that have a proven track record, like the BaleDoneen Method of heart attack, stroke, and diabetes prevention. Esophageal cancer is the fastest growing cancer in our population and is causally related to gastroesophageal reflux disease, with or without symptoms.

I recently learned at the thirty-sixth annual Esophageal and Foregut Disease Meeting, led by Dr. Steve DeMeester, that we have simple tests, commercially available, that can be administered in five minutes in the office of a family physician that can identify patients with a pre-malignant or malignant lesion that precedes the development of adenocarcinoma of the esophagus, a devastating cancer with a five-year survival rate of only 19 percent. We now possess the scientific understanding and technology to prevent reflux-related esophageal cancer, but we're still doing a miserable job of identifying those individuals at risk and of implementing effective treatment and surveillance strategies. This is related to the true lack of understanding of this complex disease by physicians. Nothing substitutes for the time the physician can spend with the patient directly or for developing innovative, individualized programs of health and wellness, but the current model of payment and care in primary care, and for that matter, in all medical specialties, does not allow for such forward thinking that would get the physician off the assembly line. In fact, medical practice is moving away from individualized care to that of population or "cookbook" medicine, meaning to apply the same diagnostic and treatment strategies to all types of patients. This is a tragic strategic error in thinking of many of our thought leaders in medicine and especially primary care.

Here lies the problem today in Medicine. Physicians that are scientific in their approach to your care are not being fostered. They're actually discouraged, especially by those leading primary care nationally. In years past, physicians committed themselves to be lifelong learners and scientists. Physicians were educated and trained to be critical thinkers. They possessed the skills and ability to search and evaluate the medical literature, and they had a basic understanding of the scientific method and what good study methodology entailed. They also developed pattern recognition in their patients over a lifetime of practice. They learned to observe a group of signs and symptoms and clinical findings on physical exam. This resulted in accurate diagnoses and effective treatments. Physicians were taught to treat the patient, not a laboratory value or diagnostic test result. And they learned not to be tyrannized by the evidence, much less depend on someone else telling them what a study said. They weren't expected to regurgitate a predetermined synopsis of the research and practice the way they were told by a so-called expert, which is robotic and mindless vs. analytical thinking based on the patient value system, the evidence and the doctor's education and clinical experience.

This is called "cookbook medicine", and in this type of approach to diagnosis and treatment, one would *not* need a highly educated and trained physician who thinks critically and scientifically. To be honest, this cookbook approach is an insult to our great profession of medicine and to every physician who paid the price of a long, arduous, demanding, and prolonged educational process, requiring them to check their brains at the door of an evidence-based symposium, which is so common today in primary care continuing education.

This is also stifling to scientific advancement and the motivation to become a master clinician. It means that the experience of a physician really means nothing, and the job can be done just was well or better by a newly graduated doctor, which we all know, empirically, is simply false. With any trade or technology, years of experience are extremely important. In primary care, there is a continued, steep learning curve for the physician, even five to seven years after their residency training is completed. As mentioned previously, there's more evidence that primary care residency training needs to be lengthened, not shortened. One of the reasons for this is that the family medicine residency is typically shorter than many of the medical and surgical specialties. For example, many of the surgical specialties, with added laboratory years for research and specialized fellowships, can run ten years after graduating from medical school.

It's hard to believe, but I have read some so-called experts who want to further reduce the residency training of family physicians from three years to two years. How ridiculous! Instead, I would recommend lengthening it by one to two more year to shore up their full scope of chronic disease management and the institution of integrative preventative models of care. This should happen if, and only if, fairness in support and reimbursement is instituted for primary care, including pay equal to that enjoyed by our specialist colleagues. This reimbursement, then adopted by Medicare and commercial health insurances is currently determined on a yearly basis by a subcommittee of the American Medical Association called the RUC (previously defined) with primary care only having one vote. RUC has been unfair to primary care physicians since its inception and more generous in their reimbursement formula to specialists and especially those who do surgeries and procedures. This is where primary care reimbursement reform needs to take place and become on par with that of our specialist colleagues!

Today, young physicians gather in person or on the internet to hear summaries and conclusions by a few in their respective fields of specialty on varies topics in medicine. They're not being challenged to think critically and evaluate the evidence based on their education and experience. They're not applying their knowledge to the individual patient but to populations of patients. These so-called experts in evidence-based medicine are essentially deciding not only how doctors practice but often who lives and who dies. These presenters rarely present the methodology, which is critical to the conclusions drawn. Many of these experts are not practicing physicians but full-time teachers. You know the old saying, "If you can't do, then teach." Young physicians today are essentially told what to think, what to conclude, and what to do without forming their own opinions. In contrast, physicians should perform as independent patient centric physicians, openly challenging conclusions drawn based on the whole of the evidence and their clinical experiences over the years of practice.

In view of this common party line thinking (i.e., group think) and interpreting the evidence, it's not surprising that physicians can be replaced by non-physicians, like nurse practitioners (NPs) and physician assistants (PAs). These are the ones compensating for the growing physician primary care shortage. Sometimes they are hired just because the hospital can save money by paying them a slightly lower salary than primary care doctors. In fact, the way the medical-industrial complex is directing medicine, it won't be long before artificial intelligence will take over mass amounts of patient diagnosis and care, and we will see the judgement and wisdom of the experienced and learned scientific physician carved into little pieces among many health care professionals. Medicine will continue to be non-coordinated, fragmented, impersonal, and population based.

If you don't believe me, try being a primary care physician and inviting hospice to come in and help manage your patient. They'll usually abide by the letter of the law but figure they know better than the doctor. They generally take over the care because they have the end-of-life expertise, even though you may have taken care of the patient for twenty years or longer and you're the patient's doctor. Some medical thought leaders consider this best end of life care according to a profit/loss ratio. They'd rather do this than what's best for the individual patient and their family.

I received the educational grant two years running at Mayo Clinic, Scottsdale. I shared this prestigious award with two of my neurology colleagues at Mayo Clinic, Scottsdale (Drs. Wingerchuck and Demaerschalk, in 2001 and 2002), to instruct all our medical students, residents, and fellows in the methodology of evidence-based medicine. This methodology was first introduced at McGill University, in Canada, in the 1970s and 1980s, only to catch fire in the early 2000s in the US. In our course, we taught that the physician scientist should never be tyrannized by the evidence. Unfortunately, this is exactly what has happened nationwide. No longer is it fashionable for the physician to come to his or her own conclusions on a medical topic or the medical literature or to personalize it to an individual patient. However, Dr. David Sackett, from McMaster University, said, "Without clinical expertise, practice becomes tyrannized by external evidence, for even excellent external evidence may be inapplicable or inappropriate for an individual patient. On the other hand, without correct best external evidence, practice becomes rapidly out of date, to the detriment of patients." This is an important point, which I made years ago at the Mayo Clinic medicine grand rounds in the early 2000s.

As you read on in this book, I'm hoping to convince you that the membership primary care model—which you, as the patient, participate in helping to fund, just like you do with your health insurance plan—will be the best medical and financial decision you make in your life. Your participation in this model should result in you living a long and prosperous life, free from physical, mental, and spiritual disabilities that, when present, can decrease the quality of life to a point that it creates hopelessness, making life not worth living.

With this book, I'm pulling back the covers on all that has held back my great specialty, family medicine, from being in a position to help you. I want you to see how our hands have been tied and how membership primary care will change your life, your health, and health care course for the rest of your life.

Chapter 4

WHAT IS A MEMBERSHIP-BASED FAMILY MEDICINE PRACTICE MODEL?

Membership has its privileges.
—Slogan made famous by American Express

Membership family medicine is available, affordable, and it's worth every penny and more to have a Marcus-Welby-type experience with all the modern technology and ease of communicating with your doctor. This new model of practice is patient centric above all else. The emphasis is on early identification of root causes of disease and aging, and on modifying them before the disease manifests. You have a doctor and staff that knows you by name for life, and a medical home serving you. A membership-based primary care practice is generally a solo family physician or general internist who charges the patient a yearly membership fee. The average is $150 a month, $450 a quarter, or $1,800 a year, but it can range from $600 to $10,000 per year. This fee is for services far beyond what's covered by Medicare or commercial health insurance plans. If a patient can afford a smart phone, internet service, gourmet coffee daily, and other monthly utility bills, he or she can afford the average cost of a membership primary care physician, and unlike the other services, this has the potential of saving their lives, adding health and longevity, and going a long way to preventing financial ruin. You can see that this additional cost is obtainable for most working adults. It boils down to the question of how much they value their health over other things, which are often around discretionary entertainment. This is where the hard decision is made. The best promotion of membership practice is when the patient experiences the major inadequacies of routine, underfunded, underperforming, insurance-based primary care, and the lack of coordination and navigation through specialty medicine and complex hospital systems.

We've structured our additional services around complementary and alternative medicine (CAM) services and programs such as cutting-edge programs for the prevention of heart attack, stroke, and diabetes. This is what membership primary care covers that is not covered by health insurance. Remember that Medicare and commercial health insurances don't generally cover these or any other preventative services, but rather a disease-based insurance coverage. And we have advanced expertise in utilizing medicinal-grade nutritional supplementation complementary to lifestyle changes and medicine and surgery. The integration of these two phenomenally successful CAM programs adds value to our membership offering. We see better outcomes for the patient when they follow the recommended therapies. Tom Blue, a national thought leader in membership medicine, would categorize this approach as "root cause medicine."

This results in the physician spending much more time and focus on providing CAM services to the patient members, because the number of patients in the doctor's panel has been reduced to around 10 percent of his or her original panel size. It gives the family physician more time face to face with the patient than the average seven minute visit. With this extra time, the physician is now able to evaluate and treat not only a single medical or health problem but the whole person—body, mind, and spirit. Many older patients have twenty or more ongoing chronic medical conditions and many need to be addressed multiple times per year. Taking advantage of the unique training and ability of the family physician and his or her full scope of practice helps to lower the overall cost of the care for that patient, with better outcomes.

In the current, fast-paced model of care, the patient, government, and commercial insurance companies are paying twice or more for health care than the next developed country in the world pays. However, this is *not* to primary care which receives only five percent of all the healthcare dollars spent in the US. Yet for all the money spent on healthcare in the US, one report concludes that among the developed nations of the world, the US ranks thirty-seventh in the quality of the health of our citizens. In my mind, healthy lifestyle, including reduction of stress and quality and freshness of food, has a lot to do with this, as well as available clean water and clean air. France and Italy are at the top of this list of countries in the world with the best health. This will be further discussed in chapter 8, which discusses medicinal-grade nutritional supplementation.

One can see that in 2020, and with the COVID pandemic still ongoing into the fall and winter, exploding in January 2021, we are at a tipping point for radical, out-of-the-box thinking to reform health care in the US. Analysis by the American Academy of Family Physicians in late April 2020 forecast furloughs, layoffs, and reduced office hours that translated to 58,000 fewer primary care physicians, and as many as 725,000 fewer nurses and other medical staff in their offices.

In 2018, there were about 223,000 primary care doctors in the US. The projected loss would be up to 26 percent of all our primary care physicians. We need a one-to-one ratio of primary care physicians to all other specialists in our country to have a cost-effective health care system. If we suffer this loss, that will reduce us to one-to-four ratio of primary care to specialty medicine in the US. One can see that our situation in primary care is critical, and something major will have to be done to save it. Waiting for the government and the medical-industrial complex to fix the situation can be unsettling, and, realistically, the changes we want them to make will likely never come, but you have a choice—an immediately achievable opportunity to locate and join a membership primary care practice as described in this book.

Chapter 5

Expanding Availability of Membership Family Physicians Is the Key to Health Care Reform.

Setbacks lead to innovation and renewed achievement.
—John Condry, famous educator

The largest health care crisis in America is not that every man, woman, and child is not insured. It's that primary care physicians, the great diagnosticians and patient educators, are becoming an endangered species. Primary care physicians, in the past, have been responsible for seeing two-thirds of all outpatient visits in the US. Currently, primary care physicians have dwindled to only twenty percent of our entire physician workforce in the US. Not only do we lack sufficient primary care physicians, but they only receive around five percent of all health care dollars spent. In contrast, hospitals receive over one-third of all dollars spent on health care. So, we can conclude that a country can't run vibrant and effective primary care services with so few doctors working in primary care and with such little economic support from the medical-industrial complex.

As pointed out by the late Dr. Barbara Starfield, in the last half century, our country has not put sufficient emphasis on a good infrastructure of primary care. She said "Everywhere in the world but the US, primary care is most of the care, for most of the people, most of the time." She goes on to point out that a lot of subspecialty care is not necessary if you have good primary care. She asserts that for health care reform to be successful in the US, the system must focus on providing more primary care to more people. It's this excuse, already not having enough primary care doctors, that the American Academy of Family Physicians use to not support and foster membership primary care. As pointed out, membership primary care seeks to take care of hundreds of patients rather than thousands. But I contend you are not fostering good primary care when you can only spend seven minutes face to face with your patient. They have not identified or fought for their members (i.e., Family Doctors) to have adequate time and reimbursement in patient care. I am not the first, nor will I be the last to point this out to our Academy only to land on a deaf ear. The rapid growth and expansion of urgent care facilities are siphoning off the easy, single, acute medical problems away from primary care doctors. These urgent care facilities have gone so far as to call themselves Primary Care. This is the case of a Walgreens Drug store close to my office in Scottsdale. The primary care doctor is left with handling the sickest and most complex patients which require so much more time than a simple single self-limited medical problem such as a viral respiratory infection. Before the advent of urgent care facilities, primary care doctors would intersperse these acute simple problem patients between more difficult cases to gain back time that would be shifted to the patients requiring more time. That is what I mean by easier patients. For the most part this is less available as many of the younger generation prefer the ease of getting in and out of an urgent care facility to a longer wait for an appointment with their primary care doctor and sitting in his or her waiting room up to one hour or longer as the doctor is often running behind. Primary care doctors simply need more time and much fewer patients in their panels such as a maximum of 500, *not* 5,000 active patients to truly be the navigator and coordinator of the patient's care. Dr. Starfield and several other thought leaders discuss this in an on-line video recorded in December 2008 *New England Journal of Medicine* roundtable presentation. Dr. Starfield goes on to say that we know from the evidence that if you don't deal with people's problems, they're much less likely to get better. Family medicine takes a whole person approach to the patient's biopsychosocial problems, which no other specialty in medicine is trained to do. As she indicates, it must be comprehensive, instead of referral-based, and it must be coordinated. The membership primary care model does it the best and provides the family physician time to get it done right.

Remember that health insurance is *not* health care. The idea that government, medical societies, such as the AMA and for-profit health insurance providers, will make the best decisions for the care of our patients and in support of primary care is sketchy, based on their track record. And these "theoretical physicians" have ideas for reimbursing primary care physicians on value outcomes. Their metric of value has become more and more cumbersome to the doctor and has led to the demise of patient care. These are not good reflections of improved care.

They are also often self-serving to the medical-industrial complex and are based on everything that is wrong with medicine and not patient-centric, certainly not doctor-centric. When primary care physicians are surveyed, they always list regulatory affairs and recording of metrics as their number one reason for burn-out and frustration with the practice of medicine. You might think it would be salaries and their income, which is usually last on their list, because these doctors really care about their patients and their health, and they put themselves last, unlike some others who work in the medical field but do not delivery direct patient care. You might be surprised to know that for every doctor who delivers patient care, there are at least 5 other workers in healthcare who push pencils or type on computers and do not deliver healthcare, telling us doctors (who took the Hippocratic Oath) what we can and can't do in the practice of medicine. Something seems desperately wrong with this picture.

A great example of this overreach by the medical-industrial complex is to tell doctors they're incapable of evaluating the whole of the experience and research with hydroxychloroquine use in early COVID infections in high-risk patients and instructing pharmacies nationwide not to fill doctors' prescriptions. In my forty-five years of medicine, pharmacy, surgical research, and teaching medical students and residents how to conduct research and evidence-based medicine, I have never seen anything more politically motivated than the withholding of this generally safe, cheap, and generic drug from our valued citizens with early COVID infections. There was no other potentially effective treatment other than to recover on your own or go into phase 2 of the COVID infection, which results in severe illness and, too often, in death by cytokine storm. There will be more on this in chapter 11.

The point is that not only is the family physician an endangered species, but those that do remain are working for the man, meaning currently more than half of all physicians work for a health care system and are not working for you directly, the patient. It's time that you, as the patient, seek out and demand a membership primary care physician. Having a membership primary care physician could result in a life-or-death situation for you and we choose life.

I propose that we start by rebuilding our health care system from the foundation up and that we rebuild primary care as the corner stone of a lean, efficient, and effective US health care delivery system, like we find in the rest of the world. And I'm attempting to make a strong argument that we have the model, although currently underutilized in the nation, with only about 20,000 membership primary care doctors practicing in the US as of 2019, per *Concierge Medicine Today*. This model is most effective and is doctor-patient driven for both the management and prevention of disease. It results in measurably significant better outcomes and health care dollar savings. For example, what if we could prevent, stabilize, and reverse the underlying disease that causes heart attacks, strokes, and even diabetes. This technology and methodology have existed for over twenty years, and I have seen the outstanding results of such programs as the BaleDoneen Method, and I've been practicing it since January 2014. Any family physician or internist can learn this basic methodology in a two-day course, if and only if they've the time to take the course, organize it in their practice, and have the time to spend with the patient and get comfortable with this unique approach to arteriology and commit to staying updated in this method. The method is dynamic, which means the primary care physician needs continuing ongoing updates, education, and review of published studies in the field.

You can see that, for the primary care physician, time is the missing link. In a sense, we've been betrayed by our "leaders" and teachers in family medicine. We've been told to believe that primary care could be delivered effectively through of brief office visit (7 minutes on the average). Family medicine is broad and deep and wide and requires special talents to multi-task and manage a whole host of areas of medicine. It's often the older medical students who have other significant work and life experiences, who are most attracted to family medicine. They desire and feel confident to take on the role of the fully practicing and functional independent family physician. They are required to know a lot about so many different areas of medicine and about life in general to serve the patient and their families as their health care advocate.

To demonstrate how clueless some of the so-called thought leaders in family medicine are (just my opinion), some have suggested we should further shorten our limited three years of residency training, which is the shortest among all surgical and medical specialty residency training periods. If family medicine was more attractive to medical students with a better work environment, equal pay for equal work and equal respect to our other medical specialties, with the recommendations made in this book, I believe medical students would be willing spend one to two additional years in training. This extra year or two in training would allow time to learn the scientific method, the skills to coordinate and navigate all of the patient's health and wellness experiences. Extending family medicine residency training takes the argument away from the AMA RUC to not pay primary care doctors equal to other medical specialists because of shorter residency training. The better trained primary care doctor with a four or five year residency would have the knowledge and experience to manage all aspects of the patient's care and be recognized as the captain or leader of the patient's healthcare team. A system we have already discussed as stated by the late Dr. Barbara Starfield.

This would allow the time to teach more CAM and business skills so that doctors could be effective in independent practice. It would also raise the reimbursement and bring respect back to the specialty of family medicine. Then there would be the same competition for family medicine as for the training programs in some of the surgical specialties. The weak family medicine training programs would have to improve or close.

One other thing: it's time that family medicine training, our academy, and all of academia in medicine be open to doctors who embrace a more conservative world view, as it has been to those who hold liberal ideas and values. We need diversity in ideology as much as we do in ethnicity and backgrounds. Free speech and the debate of ideas in the public square have made America great and free. It is in our DNA and in the foundation of this great country. Otherwise, you continue to close out fifty percent or more of your practicing family physicians to policy making, leadership, and teaching positions. I promise you that the bias is real, active, and present, as I have experienced it firsthand. Those doctors in teaching positions typically are given the time and resources to serve in these positions, whereas practicing family physicians are working on such thin financial margins and are so overworked with patient care that they do care but simply don't have the time or resources to serve on the state and national organizations that set professional policies. So, the more conservative and practical ideas and voices are never heard from a high percentage of practicing family physicians.

Finally, family medicine residents must move out of the academic teaching centers and specialist offices and academia exclusively and log significant hours with the independent, community-based family physicians that are working in the community and rural settings. These doctors have developed forward thinking ideas and concepts that work in the real world of the practice of medicine. It was these experiences I had in some of my medical school rotations with community and rural primary care doctors who were masterful at confronting real world patient centric problems, that greatly influenced me to go into family medicine. Medical academia and teaching hospitals decide what to teach, which is often not what is needed in the community the family physician will serve after residency training.

Someone must pay the physician for his or her time. For a professional, whether an attorney, CPA, or physician, our large numbers of years of education, training, and experience are the most valuable commodity we have, and we should be reimbursed more directly for our time. We should also be paid directly by the patient, rather than by an expensive insurance policy. Yet the medical-industrial complex has asked us to give it away free of charge, especially in primary care. This is crazy and does not even make common sense. The Bible tells us that the worker is worthy of his wages (Matt. 10:10, Luke 10:7, I Tim. 5:18). Most doctors are extremely charitable, yet they resent being required to work for free so that commercial insurances can make profits hand over fist, including multimillion-dollar salaries paid to the CEOs and large dividends to shareholders and administrative leadership. In addition, many hospitals are nonprofit systems, are tax exempt, and often have well-funded foundations in their communities which further financially support their costs. Health insurance companies had a financial windfall during 2020 with the COVID pandemic, because patients' utilization of services fell off steeply, but the cost of their policies continue to rise ever year. There are simply too many powerful vested interest groups in medicine that keep the system stuck. They refuse to change because they have too much to lose.

One could argue that primary care physicians have one of the hardest, and most time-consuming and labor-intensive, work of all physician specialists. Yet we're paid at the lowest rates of all our physician colleagues. We also have the highest rates of dissatisfaction and burn-out of all physicians—as much as 50 percent. Contrast this with the high-paying and very narrowly focused specialty of dermatology. Dermatology is primarily procedure based. Primary care is primarily a cognitive based-practice, meaning they're using their medical and scientific skills to diagnose, manage, and treat the patient, while a dermatologist is freezing, performing biopsies, and surgically cutting out a lesion from the skin most of the time. The dermatologist is paid far more and can see far more patients in a day. They're also the most satisfied and happiest specialists in all of medicine, with few after-hour or weekend calls from patients. Let's face it, they don't have to worry much about the patient after hours or on weekends. They don't have to deal with the extremely sick that require ER and hospitalization or even care coordination. Their work is highly focused on skin, and even their required coding and the use of electronic medical records is so much easier than for a family physician, who is coding from A to Z with the 68,000 ICD-10 codes.

Nearly always, when referring a patient to a dermatologist, I must request office notes and pathology reports so I can review them and add to my patient's medical record. It appears standard for dermatology not to identify or send copies of their visits to the referring primary care physician. This is likely due to their high patient volume. Not sending their notes significantly reduces their overhead costs, to the detriment of patient care coordination. Contrast that with a primary care doctor that must know not only dermatology but over twenty other medical and surgical specialties. Because the scope of practice of the primary care doctor is so broad, everything is always becoming more complex and challenging, from coding the correct diagnosis to having a working knowledge of the various specialty fields to the medical documentation of the visit, as the science and business of medicine advances. The primary care physician is also seeing many patients in the office who have lists of symptoms. In seven minutes, they must make at least a differential diagnosis and may need to order testing to further work up these presenting symptoms and/or refer to the correct specialists.

Although interesting, the family physician often gets a patient who hasn't yet had a diagnoses or workup. Meanwhile, a specialist may at least have some workup and a preliminary diagnosis and is not starting from scratch. You can see it's nearly impossible to provide quality care when a primary care physician is taking care of 2,000 to 5,000 patients in the practice panel. Such a doctor has limited time to see each patient in the office and even less time to review all the patient's medical records and abstract the patient chart fully. In this situation, you're lucky if the doctor even remembers your name on repeat visits.

You, the patient, can change all of this by joining a membership practice, because the primary care doctor has reduced his panel of patients by up to 90 percent. Our leadership in family medicine has been puzzled by this. They say, "How can you justify this when we already have such a shortage of primary care physicians?" I say, "How can you justify the current model of care, which has driven many our workhorse primary care doctors out of practice due to shear exhaustion and frustration? This has created such an ineffective model of care for our valued patients." The current model of care for primary care is built on a faulty foundation, and therefore we're going extinct and why our health care system is ridiculously expensive, dysfunctional, and fragmented.

The key to transformation of primary care and overall health care reform in the US is to focus on teaching and training family physicians to think critically, be able to work independently, and be adequately reimbursed in their private practice so they can limit their patient panels to no more than 500 patients. As the Bible says, we can't serve two masters, God, and money (Matt. 6:24, Luke 16:13). Primary care physicians must remain independent so they can serve the patient and not the system they work for. Often two hundred patients can be enough to keep one independent primary care physician plenty busy, especially if they're nearing or past retirement age. This will provide them significantly more time to see the patient in the office. This can be a minimum of thirty to sixty minutes for routine appointments and up to two-hour appointments for physicals combined with chronic disease management and disease prevention and new patient establishing appointments.

The membership primary care model does all of this and more and establishes the physician with the resources to pay him or her for their valuable time. Time is valuable to the doctor, but more so to the patient. It may initially seem like a hurdle for the patient to pay a yearly membership fee, but there's an adage that how much we're willing to pay for something shows how much we value it. Paying for health insurance is paying for something for the future, and the need for such can vary. In some ways, the unhealthier a patient is, the more value they receive from their insurance. In this arrangement, there is no motivation to be healthy, and most insurance companies do *not* want to invest in the patient's long-term health and wellness. After all, insurers are extremely nearsighted and figure the patient may move on to a different plan next year.

On the other hand, the primary doctor-patient relationship is one that is hopefully long term, and the goal is for the patient to get healthier and healthier as each year passes. The patient has a dog in the fight, and it's worth it to pay for this unique and valuable member patient relationship with their membership primary care physician. In addition, they have the added piece of mind that if they have an emergency, they can reach their doctor at any time by phone. Contrast that with trying to get a hold of your insurance-based doctor after hours and often not getting called back (just my general observation). I know this to be true because patients will call me and get an answer when they can't get ahold of their specialist after business hours. It didn't used to be that way, years ago. Over the past decade or two, doctors in general are having increased demand by government and insurers for non-patient related activity, documentation, and prior approvals. In addition, docs are frustrated with everyone interfering in this sacred trust relationship with the doctor-patient relationship, malpractice out of control, reimbursement for physicians low in comparison to those profiting so heavily from patient illnesses and suffering, and a general lack of respect, docs in general are less motivated to be committed to extra work after hours such as taking calls from the patient.

The patient craves this personalized time with the primary physician. They want their family physician to know them on a personal level and understand their needs and wants and desires for their health care and wellness. They want their family physician to walk with them on their health care recovery road and journey for life. And they certainly want their doctor to know their name without having to check their chart each time. You should have a doctor who knows you by name for life. You may not need a particular specialist for life, but you absolutely need your family medicine physician over your lifetime.

Chapter 6

AN INTEGRATED FAMILY PHYSICIAN IS ESSENTIAL IN THE TWENTY-FIRST CENTURY TO A SUCCESSFUL MEMBERSHIP PRACTICE

The whole is greater than the sum of its parts.
—Aristotle (384 BC–322 BC)

And this is the reason why the cure of many diseases is unknown to the physicians of Hellas, because they are ignorant of the whole, which ought to be studied also: for the part can never be well unless the whole is well.
—Socrates (470 BC–399 BC)

An integrated family medicine practice is one that practices the full scope of traditional or allopathic medicine. This means your family physician has generally graduated from college after four years and then must take a rigorous medical entrance exam before being selected to attend one of around 154 MD accredited medical schools in the US. In my case, I was thirty-five when I entered Creighton University Medical School, in Omaha, Nebraska, in 1990.

They picked around a hundred students out of 10,000 applications for my class. Most medical students who were at the top of their college class soon find out that they were a big fish in a small pond. Now, in medical school, they're a little fish in a big pond. In other words, the average medical student has an IQ of 120 (the average in the general population is 100), and they have grades that approach or are at 4.0. They've already had unusual life experiences that distinguish them from the other 9,900 applicants that were not accepted. In my case, I had achieved the doctor of pharmacy degree (PharmD) eleven years earlier. I had also finished a rigorous two-year post-PharmD residency at the University of Kentucky Medical Center, in Lexington, Kentucky, working over a hundred hours per week for two straight years in the hospital setting and serving as an associate professor of surgery and pharmacy and director of surgical research during the 1980s, having been promoted and tenured at Creighton University School of Medicine.

After finishing Medical School in 1994, I was awarded the doctor of medicine (MD) degree. Like 99 percent of medical school graduates, I went on to serve in a post-MD residency training program for three years, serving my last year as chief resident at In His IMAGE Family Medicine Residency Program, in Tulsa, OK. My training included an opportunity to travel to Ghana, West Africa, twice to serve as a Christian medical missionary to the underserved. I did everything from speaking in their two medical schools, to seeing patients in rural clinics, to taking care of sick patients in the mission's hospital, to preaching the Gospel of Jesus Christ in churches and on dirt-floor gatherings in the bush through a translator and expressing my talent of classically trained singing.

After all of this, I would later learn that some of our physician "leaders" in my professional academy and physician administrators on our hospital staff (who we affectionately refer to as "the suits") would tell us that we were not good enough. They contrived further arbitrary nonsensical quality measures that we had to achieve in order to function adequately and to compete with our specialist colleagues. It was ridiculous then and ridiculous now. Dr. Starfield and I have made the argument that family physicians are more than adequately trained and have a unique practice ethos that separates them from other specialists in the field of medicine. We are uniquely gifted; therefore, "a whole person approach for the whole family" is the tag line of my practice. In other words, your family doctor serves as your medical home and the navigator of the health care journey. This would be true, but only if they had the time, a more manageable patient panel size, and fair reimbursement for their time and overhead.

In order to maximize the justification and utilization of the membership model as the most effective model for the family physician can use to increase time with the patient, coordinate, and navigate all of the patient's health care and be reimbursed, your personal doctor needs to take one more step that is not being taught in most medical schools. He or she needs to become an integrated family physician.

An integrated physician is well grounded in traditional or allopathic medicine. In addition, the integrated physician adds practice attributes and specific programs that prevent and reverse disease. He or she ask the questions beyond just diagnosis and treatment, such as what is the root cause of this medical disorder and is it grounded in the health of the body, or mind, or spirit of the patient. How do these set of symptoms relate to all organ systems of the body and where do they originate. It is whole-person medicine, and the physician can apply it by individualizing and integrating the patient's lifestyle, medications, surgery, and medical-grade nutritional supplements and hormones. Depending on the interest of the family physician, it adds to his or her toolbox of offerings. Either the doctor can practice these technologies or refer the patient to a health care professional who does. These would include but not be limited to functional medicine, acupuncture, chiropractors, and many others that fall under the broad category of complementary and alternative medicine (CAM). To the integrated family physician, having CAM added to his or her tool box complements the ability of all the traditional medical specialties of traditional MD medicine and provides the basis for blending Medicare and commercial health care insurance reimbursements with out-of-pocket patient costs both for the medical membership, further CAM lab testing, and services not routinely covered by third-party payers. It is the best of both worlds and the health care payments are shared between traditional payers and the patients directly. More on this in chapters 9 and 10.

Membership medicine is the future of medicine, in my opinion. It allows a doctor to practice root-cause health care by allowing for longer appointments to better get to know their patients and treat them in the context of their beliefs and health care goals (biopsychosocial). Membership medicine provides the physician with the time and resources to also practice integrative medicine.

Chapter 7

HEART ATTACKS AND STROKES ARE PREVENTABLE: THE BALEDONEEN METHOD IS A PREMIER INTEGRATED MEMBERSHIP PRACTICE

Every year, approximately 785,000 Americans suffer a first heart attack. And 470,000 who've already had one or more heart attacks have another one. The scary thing is that 25 percent of all heart attacks happen silently, without clear or obvious symptoms.

—Dr. Chauncey Crandall,
chief of the cardiac transplant program at
Palm Beach Cardiovascular Clinic in Florida

Heart attack, stroke, and diabetes remain the primary drivers of health care costs, disability, and death. Cardiovascular disease remains the leading cause of death and disability for both men and women in the United States. Every twenty to thirty seconds, someone in the US has a heart attack or stroke. Each year more than 2,000,000 Americans have a heart attack or stroke, and more than forty percent of them, or 800,000 people, will die of that event. Cardiovascular disease remains the number one cause of death in the US.

Medical costs and loss of productivity approach $450 billion per year. The costs of heart attacks and strokes are projected to triple annually over the next twenty years, when adjusted for inflation. Taking a proactive approach such as managing the risk of heart attack, stroke, and diabetes has shown to be effective starting up to twenty years prior to the onset of the disease or a life threatening cardiovascular event. Obviously, we can find the early beginnings of these diseases twenty years before they are often found in a traditional medicine approach.

Current strategies for addressing the burden of cardiovascular disease have stalled out at approximately a thirty percent reduction in morbidity and mortality over the last twenty years. A new paradigm is needed to address many patients who will go on to experience major adverse cardiovascular events including death. The BaleDoneen Method provides an evidence-based approach to the prevention of heart attacks and strokes and represents the premier integrated medical program among all my offerings. Currently, it's only being practiced within a membership model due to the time required.

Fully implemented, this approach provides primary and secondary prevention of heart attacks and ischemic strokes. This has enormous ramifications for elimination of mortality and morbidity caused by the number one and number two causes of death in the US. It's also noteworthy that fifty-one percent of all cancers can be prevented by this proactive approach to healthy arteries. Just this one organized method of care could have an enormous impact in the US on patient suffering and death and on rising and out-of-control health care expenditures. In addition, this approach has been proven to prevent diabetes, thus it also reduces the burden of dementia and renal dialysis. What tremendous impact this would have on our health care system if adopted as the standard of care as it should be.

Currently, the standard of care diagnostic vascular studies emphasize flow obstruction or arterial luminal narrowing rather than a search for the presence and characterization of plaque and the presence and degree of endothelial inflammation, the common pathway to the development of unstable arterial plaque. The two leading factors, endothelial inflammation and oxidative stress, are thought to facilitate the pathogenesis and progression of atherosclerotic changes. They're the primary drivers of plaque rupture or tear. This is what causes serious and deadly cardiovascular events, not slow progressive blockage, as thought by most of the public. Prediabetes, a condition which precedes diabetes, is present and contributing to more than seventy percent of stroke and heart attack victims. Assessing multiple advanced biomarkers of vascular inflammation has been shown to have the potential to reduce our national health care costs by 15 percent, or $450 billion annually.

Can heart attacks and strokes be prevented? They absolutely can and should be. But the practice of medicine is slow to change and adopt new ideas and concepts. Practicing the status quo is always easier, especially if it means change will cause financial loss by our stakeholders. It typically takes eighteen to twenty years after the introduction of a new idea in medicine before it gets broad acceptance and common utilization in day-to-day practice. Heart attacks are the top cause of mortality and morbidity in the US, and, sad to say, there is so much more money to be made by heart specialists and hospitals and the medical-industrial complex in treating than preventing this ever so common disease, which snuffs out lives, often prematurely, and frequently leaves patients as cardiac cripples or with significant permanent neurological deficits after strokes. They are dependent on round-the-clock, full-time caregivers.

One of my mentors in medicine and surgery, Dr. Tom R. DeMeester, pointed out that there's something morally wrong with individuals and corporations excessively profiting on the backs of sick and suffering patients. Dr. DeMeester is a pioneer and a legend in the field of foregut pathophysiology and surgery. I have learned so much from him. In other words, he specialized in the pathophysiology of the esophagus, stomach, and duodenum. He has advanced our understanding and the science of gastroesophageal disease (GERD) and esophageal cancer (adenocarcinoma of the distal esophagus from GERD) as much as any physician-surgeon scientist in my lifetime. He taught us the disease's mechanisms in the 1970s and 1980s, and those teachings have withstood the test of time and are still true and relevant in the 2020s. We stand at the doorway of eliminating esophageal cancer, a dreadful and often terminal disease, but it will take the involvement of primary care doctors participating in generalized screening and appropriate patient selection for further evaluation and treatment by gastroenterologists and foregut surgeons.

The continually updated BaleDoneen Method of heart attack and stroke prevention rapidly adopts the latest findings presented in peer-reviewed publications into clinical practice. This keeps physicians and other clinicians on the leading edge of prevention. This method uses a team approach, in which medical and dental clinicians work together to save lives and with optimal care. Drs. Bale and Doneen recently published a landmark paper—the first to identify a new, treatable cause of cardiovascular disease, which is the presence of high-risk oral bacterial pathogens from periodontal or endodontal disease. Periodontal disease affects many adults over the age of thirty, many of whom are unaware that they harbor a serious oral infection that can directly cause arterial plaque.

The downside of this preventable inflammatory disease is unnecessary death and needless suffering, and it has cost our country and the world outrageously. The US spends around 17.7 percent of our gross domestic product on health care, and this pushes our national debt to (at the time of the writing of this book, during the COVID pandemic) $28 trillion and growing, with more bailouts planned. In the United States, only the federal government does not have to balance its budget. This seems to many of us unwise, unfair, and reckless, and it can lead to out-of-control inflation. This is a national security issue. This spending needs to be stopped through a constitutional amendment and term limits on Congress. We are mortgaging the futures of our children and grandchildren, including my ten children, grandchildren, and great grandchild.

Focusing on the health of the arteries has many benefits in preventing the two catastrophic cardiovascular events from which patients can either die or suffer devasting disability. There is many secondary benefits of preventing or reversing type two diabetes mellitus, which is currently the scourge on our adult and children populations. It's also the disease that's bankrupting our countries' health care economy.

The BaleDoneen Method of heart attack and stroke prevention has been taught and practiced now for over twenty years. This method focuses on identifying root causes of atherosclerotic disease, reversing these causes, and quantifying and reducing the level of arterial inflammation so that plaque present in the arteries begins to stabilize and eventually completely calcify. Fully calcified plaque does not rupture, whereas plaque rupture is the cause of major cardiovascular events. Does it not make sense to discover those individuals that have plaque in their arteries and the level of inflammation above and beyond just those patients that have already had a heart attack or stroke. Even in those who have had a previous heart attack and who are carefully following the current standard of care, fifty percent of these will have a second heart attack, and fifty percent of these will die. This is unfortunate and unnecessary.

They say it takes about twenty years for a new idea to take hold after it's introduced into medicine, so I hope we're getting near a tipping point and that our family physicians, general internists, and cardiologists will move away from arterial flow obstruction as their focus and onto the presence of plaque and inflammation and root causes. Clearly, if a heart attack is occurring, the blockage caused by a clot needs to be immediately opened with angioplasty, but not in asymptomatic patients with slow plaque buildup. This is not the mechanism by which heart attacks and plaque related strokes occur.

The BaleDoneen Method represents what I consider to be one of our premium and most highly beneficial integrated programs, which has been adopted primarily in medicine by our membership family physicians and general internists. Why? Again, these integrated membership physicians have the time and interest to learn this methodology, set up the technology in their practices, and have the time to practice and teach this to their patients. The BaleDoneen Method offers a tremendous advantage of preventing the most common cause of death and disability in the US and developed nations.

In addition, it also has the same beneficial effects on microvascular disease, which destroys our end organs, such as the brain, heart, kidneys, lungs, and intestines. This is the silent killer, again, due to arterial disease in the small arteries, the arterioles, and capillaries. Recently, I heard Dr. Bale mention that in the twenty years he's practiced this methodology, not a single one of his patients receiving this method has had to be placed on kidney dialysis.

This methodology does not simply treat flow obstruction. Rather, it addresses the pathogenesis of the disease and its many root causes. It can both arrest and reverse the disease, eliminating heart attacks and ischemic strokes, and stabilizing microvascular disease.

Chapter 8

Personalized Medical-Grade Nutritional Supplements Are Critical to Health and Wellness for Most Patients

Supplementation can benefit anyone. Whether you have perfect eating habits, or you subsist off cheeseburgers and fries, adding a quality supplement can immediately provide you with better health and added protection.

—Nicholas J. Webb

Another prime example of an integrative program that fits perfectly with a membership family medicine practice is offering medical-grade nutritional supplements to our patients. In my experience, nutritional supplements are critical for patient health and wellness. Most patients don't appreciate how woefully lacking the modern diet is in critical micronutrients. Like so many conditions in medicine, nutrient deficiencies are not fully appreciated without measuring them in the body. And how and where we measure them in the body is just as important. Critical nutrients can be measured in the bloodstream, hair, urine, and saliva, but the best way to measure them every six months to a year is by a reliable and reproducible intracellular nutrient evaluation. This test reflects the actual stores of nutrients inside the 70 trillion cells that make up your physical body.

The global nutraceutical industry (i.e., dietary supplements) is an explosive growth industry, expected to rise from $209 billion in 2017 to $373 billion by 2025. In addition, a huge factor in the success of nutrient supplements is the quality and purity of them, and most patients don't really even know what to take, what brands they can trust, or all the science in and around delivering supplements in oral dosage forms. The key is to work with a physician or health care clinician that has studied the field of nutritional supplements and knows the quality product lines to recommend. It's important to stay away from companies that engage in misbranding and adulteration of the products. That's so common in many of the products sold in stores. These suboptimal products are often sold in grocery stores and drug stores in less expensive product lines.

There are many reasons why our diet is deficient in micronutrients, including vitamins, minerals, electrolytes, and antioxidants, to mention a few. So many of our patients are eating a fast food and processed diet daily, and much of our food is mass farmed, including plants and animals. There are problems with nutrient poor soil. It's not cared for or rested properly, and crops are not rotated as was done for centuries in family farming.

Instead, vegetables are often picked green, instead of being vine ripened, through which the vital nutrients come up into the produce at the end of the growing process. These whole foods are then radiated, gassed, and shipped across the country. Then they sit in our grocery store produce shelves, looking like perfect waxed fruit. The average consumer has no idea of the quality or age of the produce. They make their selection based on how it appears.

When they take home the produce and bite into it, they're often disappointed. Their tomatoes, for example, might taste like red mush. The consumer is only getting fiber and water, and the produce often lacks the hundreds, if not thousands, of micronutrients and phytonutrients that give the fruit or vegetable its delicious smells and taste.

I contend that if the consumer could smell and taste a sample of what they were purchasing from a sample tray by each produce item, it would be nearly as good as testing it in the laboratory. If it smells and tastes like it was grown in your home garden, it likely contains an abundance of healthy micronutrients and phytonutrients. Therefore, I encourage my patients to eat the colors of the rainbow and forage for organic family farmed produce, locally grown and seasonal. Organic choices are especially important in avoiding toxic pesticides, which can cause cancer. In many fruits and vegetables, these toxic chemicals soak right into the produce and are not easily washed off. You may be familiar with the term: clean fifteen and the dirty dozen. This expression refers to the produce that more easily retains chemicals and pesticides (dirty dozen) versus those fruits and vegetables that do not (clean fifteen).

One can't speak of the benefits of nutrition and the harm of micronutrient deficiencies without mentioning the role of chronic inflammation, especially in the gut. We are learning that inflammation is the driving force not only for plaque disease but for most chronic diseases, including cancer. When there is leaky gut, gut inflammation, and dysbiosis, this disrupted lining of the gut (i.e., the enterocytes that form a barrier to the gut mucosa) allows endotoxins to travel into the systemic bloodstream and even cross the blood brain barrier into the central nervous system. This leaky and inflamed gut mucosa is a breeding ground for the development of food allergies and even some autoimmune diseases.

Obese individuals often can't lose weight for several important reasons, but right at the top of the list is that they're often on fire, burning up with inflammation as their abdominal adiposity acts like a neuroendocrine organ. They are at war in their bodies, and just like in a natural war, their body is focused on fighting the war at hand and putting off other metabolic activities that would lead to better nutritional status, weight loss, reversal of chronic inflammation, and diseases, and overall improved health. Unfortunately, discussion of this topic and the role of gut health is still a new frontier, outside the focus of this book but very much a key to the successful long-term health of the patient, slowing down aging and staving off chronic disease and autoimmune diseases.

Hippocrates said, "Let food be thy medicine and medicine be thy food." Nutritional supplements work entirely differently than medication, and therefore don't directly compete with them, even though Big Pharma feels their profits are threatened by natural remedies. Medications are chemicals, with few exceptions, and our bodies were not originally programed to digest them. Yes, many medications can be miracle pills and allow patients to cope with serious diseases and live healthier and longer, especially when disease is long standing and advanced in their bodies, but we were designed to eat plants and animals, not dirt.

As a physician and pharmacologist, I feel the fact that most of us can detoxify and metabolize medications (i.e., chemicals) shows that we are wonderfully and fearfully created by the God of the universe. The all-knowing God of the Bible is a personal God. Scripture tells us He knows the number of hairs on our heads (Matt. 10:30, Luke 12:7). He knew that man would one day discover natural remedies in nature and in plants and learn to reproduce them chemically in the laboratory. God is eternal and is not confined to the dimension of time like man is.

Unfortunately, medications don't give off good downstream communication and signaling in the body. But they can cause unwanted side effects. In contrast, a high-quality medicinal-grade nutritional supplement that doesn't contain contaminants rarely causes side effects. Beware of products that don't have a good reputation. Some are adulterated with undisclosed amounts of pharmaceutical drugs or steroid compounds, likely hidden, such as weight loss products, sexual enhancement products, body building products, and feel-good and mood products. There is usually a wide therapeutic index with supplements, meaning there is a big range between the lowest and highest blood concentrations of a nutrient in the body. So, having too little is a more likely scenario than having too much, and regularly measuring levels helps us optimize these levels of key nutrients to sustain life and avoid DNA damage, chronic disease, and accelerated aging, which occurs with chronic nutrient deficiencies. This has been written about by Dr. Bruce Ames, of Berkley, CA.

Conversely, nutritional supplements support the structure and function of the body, so it takes a patient about six months of taking a supplement before they incorporate enough of it into the new cells of the body that are being formed daily to replace dying cells, until one can appreciate a physiologically expressed positive effect, and daily supplementation refills the deficient stores in the cells of our body.

Amazingly, we are finding that many of them have multiple desirable effects in the body. They have positive downstream signaling in the body and throughout our cells. For example, a natural supplement such as quercetin might have a stabilizing effect on mast cells. This, in turn, decreases symptoms of allergies and has beneficial effects on other cells and organ systems in the body, such as the cardiovascular system. Nutritional supplements act more like food than chemical medications in the body. That is why they are called dietary or nutritional supplements. This is what nutrients do, and if there were enough micronutrients in our modern-day diet, we wouldn't need to supplement them. The best way to be sure we're getting enough is to routinely check cellular levels, which reflect how much cellular stores or reserves we have in our body. Let your nutrient evaluation guide what supplements you should take, and get the advice of a membership physician who is knowledgeable in nutraceuticals to help you with this process.

Incorporation of nutraceuticals into patient care changed for the better in 1994 with the passage by Congress of the Dietary Supplement Health and Education Act (DSHEA), which not only called on the FDA to regulate dietary supplements under a separate regulation than food and medications, but to prevent the adulteration and misbranding of them, and to encourage physicians and other health care clinicians to educate their patients on the potential benefits of dietary supplements. DSHEA provides FDA with appropriate regulatory authority while still allowing consumers to have the desired access to a wide variety of affordable, high quality, safe and beneficial dietary supplement products.

I believe that nutraceuticals (i.e., vitamins and herbal supplements) are a cornerstone to the preventive health care movement. They should be combined with nutritious whole foods, which serve as antidotes to the toxic insult of our current environmental toxicities, such as unclean air, water, and processed foods filled with chemicals and preservatives. Try to eat more foods without a label, and if your food is labeled, make sure it contains only ingredients you can pronounce, and five or fewer is a good rule of thumb.

One of the more imaginative, out-of-the-box thinkers and researchers on the short-term and long-term negative effects of micronutrient deficiencies is Dr. Bruce Ames, of Berkley, California. He came up with the Ames triage theory. He points out that depending on the diet and the presence of thirty to forty key micronutrients in the soil from region to region, from time to time an individual will be deficient in one or more of these essential micronutrients. When the body receives some of the deficient micronutrient, it sends it to the most critical metabolic processes for our immediate survival and allows the cells critical for long term survival to go without. When this deficiency goes on for a long period of time, it ultimately results in breaks in the DNA and accelerates chronic diseases that cause aging, such as cancer. Clearly, this demonstrates a role of routine intracellular measurement of micronutrients and routine supplementation based on the individual patient's chronic disease states, sex, age, diet habits, and the results of the micronutrient testing. My advice, and what appears to be the consensus of most experts, is to consume a Mediterranean diet and selective supplements as needed per intracellular testing.

The membership family physician of the future will be excellent in traditional medicine and pharmacology and will have a good understanding of when intervention and surgery is the treatment of choice. He or she will also integrate multiple and useful alternative and complementary medicines, leading to early detection, wellness, and prevention. Nutrition and nutritional supplementation are already here, and patients, in many ways, are far ahead of their allopathic traditional physicians. Remember that the number one commodity needed by physician and patient alike is adequate time to work together on these high-dividend, complementary programs. Nothing substitutes fully for quality time and education provided to the patient, and only in the membership family medicine model can this be best achieved.

Chapter 9

Faith and Medicine Are Compatible and Desirable and Can be Mixed with Sensitivity and Compassion

Truth is so obscure in these times, and falsehood so established, that, unless we love the truth, we can't know it.

—Blaise Pascal (1623–1662)

In the Bible, Christ Jesus was referred to as the Physician (Matt. 5:12, Luke 5:31). He went about during his three-and-a-half year ministry on planet Earth supernaturally healing all who were sick and oppressed by the devil. As Christ's followers, we're told not to hide our light under a bushel, yet physicians, like many who work in the secular world, feel uncomfortable incorporating their faith and Christian values into the workplace and their spheres of influence. Yet turning our backs on the culture is a betrayal of our biblical mandate and our own heritage because it denies God's sovereignty over all of life.

Abraham Kuyper, the great nineteenth-century theologian who served as prime minister of Holland from 1901 to 1905, said that the dominating principle of Christian truth is not soteriological (justification by faith) but cosmological (the sovereignty of the triune God over the whole cosmos, in all its spheres and kingdoms, visible and invisible). He was a statesman, pastor, theologian, journalist, philosopher, and founder of the Free University of Amsterdam in 1880. He believed, as I do, that Christ was sent to redeem every aspect of society and that Christ's followers were left with the mandate and responsibility to complete what He initiated, notwithstanding the discipline of medicine. Christ Jesus was and is our healer and the Physician.

The separation of religion and government was never meant to exclude religion from the public square. It simply meant the government couldn't dictate the religion we had to follow, as spelled out in the Constitution. Americans wanted to avoid the tyranny they'd fled in England, where everyone had to support and be submissive to the Church of England. Even though our constitution recognizes all religions and religious freedom, the United States of America was firmly founded and grounded on biblical and Judeo-Christian principles and values, as expressed in our Constitution and Bill of Rights.

For over two millennia, Christian doctors and nurses, inspired by the example and teaching of Jesus of Nazareth, have been at the forefront of efforts to alleviate human suffering, cure disease, and advance knowledge and understanding. Christians and the Christian church have played major roles in developing and shaping the practice of medicine. Jesus Christ, who the church holds as its founder, instructed His followers to heal the sick. The early Christians were noted for caring for the sick and infirm, and Christian emphasis on charity gave rise to the development of nursing and hospitals.

In the Catholic Church, the influential Benedictine rule holds that "the care of the sick is to be placed above and before every other duty, as if indeed Christ were being directly served by waiting on them." Jesus is recorded in the New Testament as saying, "For I was hungry and you fed me, thirsty and you gave me drink. I was a stranger and you received me in your homes. Naked and you clothed me. I was sick and you took care of me, in prison and you visited me...Whatever you did for one of these least brothers of mine, you did for me" (Matt. 25:31–40).

Pagan religions seldom offered help to the sick. However, early Christians were willing to nurse the sick and feed them. The church's involvement in health care has ancient origins. The ancient Greek and Roman medicine developed solid foundations over seven centuries, creating the ideal of a union of science, philosophy, and practical medicine in the learned physician. But Greek and Roman religion did not preach of a duty to tend to the sick. Conversely, Christianity emerged into this world in the mid-first century, and from the outset they went about taking care of the sick and infirm. The disciples of Jesus were healers. Dr. Luke the evangelist, who wrote the Gospel of Luke, was a physician and a scholar and a Christ follower.

In the Graeco-Roman world, life was often cruel and inhumane. The weak and sick were despised. Abortion, infanticide, and poisoning were widely practiced. From the fourth century to present times, Christians were prominent in the building of hospitals and raising the money for them. The first large-scale hospital, with three hundred beds, was founded in AD 369 by Saint Basil of Caesarea. The advances of medical knowledge were led by Jews and Christians and are too enormous to cover in this chapter. However, it is noteworthy that the Roman Catholic Church is the largest non-government provider of health care services in the world today. They have around 18,000 clinics, 16,000 homes for the elderly, and 5,500 hospitals. It is estimated that the Church manages twenty six percent of the world's health care facilities.

As a Christian physician who believes in the marriage (not the separation) of faith and medicine, history is on my side. It's only been in this current post-modern world that there has been concern and caution about physicians and patient's discussing spirituality and the professional boundaries and potential ethical issues. Clearly, a patient's faith and spirituality often play major roles in how patients cope effectively with severe, chronic, and terminal conditions.

Some of the more recent published literature on this subject seems to be dominated by the disciplines of psychiatry and psychology. It would seem that sensitivity, compassion, and even common sense have been replaced with complexity, theory, and, to some extent, psychobabble. Most physicians today believe in God, whereas, it is estimated that only twenty-five percent of psychologists believe in God. Looking into the roots of Christianity and Dr. Sigmund Freud, Austrian neurologist and father of modern-day psychoanalysis, helps to explain why so few psychologists embrace faith in a healing God. Most do not really believe in the power of prayer or supernatural healing.

We all need mentors to follow, as few of us are ever courageous enough to explore uncharted waters and navigate a clear path for others to follow. Family physician and surgeon Dr. William Standish Reed, MD, author of *Surgery of the Soul*, to my knowledge is just that courageous pioneer for those of us Christian physicians who believed in, studied, and practiced his unique approach to the practice of medicine. Dr. Reed married his surgical and medical practice with the healing power of prayer and by the miraculous power of the Holy Spirit, in performing documented medical miracles. While in medical school at the University of Michigan, Dr. Reed wrote, "There occurred within my heart a sense that God was giving me an imperative to see if the spiritual orientation of practice could be in some way instituted in America, and hopefully, Canadian medicine in a day of increasing emphasis on science and mechanization." Dr. Reed saw his dream come to fruition in

1960 in Texas. He relocated to Tampa, Florida, in 1964, where he ran a hospital with a focus on prayer and healing, providing top surgical and medical care, often to those that were hopeless cases in traditional medical hospitals.

Ground was broken, with other medical pioneers working toward the spiritual in its consideration of providing healing to man. The writings of Alexis Carrel created a furor and a storm in medical circles. Dr. Carrel, along with Dr. Howard Kelly, of Johns Hopkins University, and Dr. Richard Cabot, of Harvard, were indeed pioneers of a new, vital, and much-needed area in the practice of medicine and surgery, looking beyond the treatment of the physical and the mental and considering deeply the spiritual in the treatment of the whole man.

Dr. Reed points out in his book, *Surgery of the Soul*, that we have made the error of believing that the psychological and the spiritual are one and the same. The Bible tells us that man has three parts: body, mind, and spirit. And a physician should be able to diagnose and treat a medical or health problem in one or all these parts of man, a term he coined whole person medicine or logo-psychosomatic medicine. He approached healing the whole person by developing a harmony between the spirit, the mind, and the body. He believes that the faith of the Christian in the Word of God and in the Lord, Jesus Christ, can effect transformation of impossible situations into possible ones, darkness and hopelessness into light and optimism, and sickness into health.

In 1734, Alexander Pope said, "As the twig is bent, so grows the tree." It was my Christian faith and commitment which led me, at age thirty-five, to enter medical school to become a physician. And it is the presence of Christ with me daily in my medical practice by the fellowship of the Holy Spirit, a gift to all believers from Christ, that helps me give more optimal care, knowledge, and wisdom to my patients. This is best illustrated in the painting by Nathan

Greene, used for the cover on this book, called *The Difficult Case*. Give me divine insight and miracles over all the learned knowledge in all the books of the world. I affectionately termed this the "G" or God factor. But realize all knowledge and revelation comes from God almighty.

After medical school, I chose a Christian family medicine residency training program in Tulsa, OK, called In His Image Family Medicine Residency Program, so I would not have to divest my faith in God while learning to be a competent family physician. Instead, the program would strengthen my faith and allow me to learn how to incorporate faith and medicine in a compassionate and sensitive way that nearly all patients would find to be caring and a comfort. In this decision I would be giving credit and glory to the God, who provided the knowledge and understanding of medical advances over the past two millennia and to His influence in so many physicians, scientists, and health care professionals whose shoulders I stand upon. I wanted to learn how to integrate faith, prayer, scripturally inspired counseling, and words of encouragement to my patients as led by the sensitivity and timing of the Holy Spirit. I want to combine my faith with that of the patient, to look to God to do the impossible (Luke 1:37). Nearly all my patients over the years, both in the US and overseas in the mission field, have welcomed and received my services as a Christian physician, with grateful hearts, desiring to be healed and made whole again through the science of medicine and the supernatural power of the Holy Spirit.

Chapter 10

HEALTH INSURANCE IS NOT HEALTH CARE

Insurance companies have killed primary care by grinding down reimbursement and compelling doctors to see more and more patients just to make a living.
—Richard M. Hannon,
Sr. V.P. of Marketing and Provider Affairs,
Blue Cross Blue Shield of Arizona

When you boil down health care to its most essential elements, it gets right back to the doctor-patient relationship. Before we had the current bulky, top-heavy, overregulated, overcontrolled, and profit-generating medical facilities, government agencies, and insurers, you had studied and well-trained individuals serving as medical physicians and surgeons, taking care of patients. Governmental decisions that seem well meaning and potentially beneficial can have unexpected and detrimental consequences, in this case to the doctor-patient relationship.

On July 30, 1965, President Lyndon B. Johnson signed into law legislation that established the Medicare and Medicaid programs. It was not until 1966 that patients began to receive these benefits. In later years, Congress expanded Medicare eligibility to younger people with permanent disabilities. This was all done with good intentions in the beginning, but the government quickly began to use it as a mechanism by which to control the practice of medicine, as the entitlement of Medicare and Medicaid currently pays for over 50 percent of all health care costs in this country, and whoever pays for the services controls the services.

Initially, this was a windfall for the physicians. Their services had guaranteed financial coverage. They didn't have to be paid in chickens and eggs by those who could not afford to pay with cash. But little by little, more and more regulations and requirements were placed on these payments, interfering with the doctor-patient therapeutic relationship. After a while, physicians had less and less control and influence in the practice of medicine.

Primary care physicians were hurt the most by this change in a time of the rapid growth in numbers and wealth of hospitals. Nonprofit hospitals were also supported with active foundations, and sub-specialization of medicine. The American Medical Association had little respect for the general practitioner and gave their full weight of support to specialists, especially those doing procedures, to receive the lion's share of the Medicare reimbursement dollars. Commercial insurances have always followed the lead of the rate setting for Medicare/Medicaid by CMS.gov (Centers for Medicare and Medicaid Services). Early on, specialists fought hard for their reimbursement via the AMA's RUC, while benevolent family physicians, who relied mostly on their cognitive skills, gratefully took whatever reimbursement was allocated to them.

Family physicians were dependent on their national organization, the American Academy of Family Physicians, to lobby for higher reimbursement, but they got into this game with too little and too late. Today, when the financial reimbursement pie is divided, hospitals do well, and many don't pay taxes because they're organized as nonprofit corporations. They receive additional funding from their strong, community-based, or even national foundations, and they receive about one third of the total reimbursement pie. That's a larger piece than even the for-profit health insurance companies and pharmaceutical companies.

The hospitals, as a group, spend more money than any other health care group lobbying congress yearly, and their CEOs and executives draw salaries higher than most other company CEOs and even university presidents. Conversely, primary care physicians, who have been responsible for seeing over two thirds of all outpatient visits, receive only around 5 percent of the health care reimbursement. This is hard to justify on any level and one of the primary reasons we have such a severe shortage of primary care physicians, the most burned out and dissatisfied specialty of medicine. Without an altruistic call to family medicine or general internal medicine, it's near impossible to get medical school graduates to choose primary care as a career choice, and never mind trying to get their sons and daughters to enter medicine as a career, when the most needed but most underfunded and under respected specialty in medicine goes year after year without transformation and reform.

You've been told, and you have believed, the greatest lie in modern health care. Your health insurance, no matter how wonderful it is, is not health care. Great health care is provided by great physicians. Remember President Obama's promise to you during his creation of Obamacare. If you like your doctor, you can keep your doctor. Health insurance is simply a means of paying for part of the health care services you receive. Long gone are the Cadillac health care policies that cover most of your health care costs. More common today are $5,000 to $10,000 in annual deductibles, and then, when the deductible is met, you're required to pay ten percent to thirty percent of the costs of services going forward.

The more a health insurance company involves themselves in providing health care and making health care decisions, which should only be made by the doctor and patient together, the poorer the quality. And often, vital tests and therapeutics are denied coverage by the health insurance company, when the patient was promised unrestricted medical care, when they were sold a less expensive healthcare policy.

In patients of Medicare age, they call these plans advantage plans, and they look attractive to seniors, but as they say, if it's too good to be true, it usually is. There is no such thing as a free lunch. There is no stronger example of this than the HMO insurance products. They're cheaper, but you're giving your insurance company the authority to decide what you can and can't receive, and it's a massive headache to your physician to try to argue and justify why a test needs to be ordered, especially when they're talking to a doctor who works for the insurance company and is often trained in an unrelated specialty area.

Patient care is hard and demanding, and some doctors seem willing to do anything to avoid patient care, such as working for an insurance company and often denying services. Remember, private insurance companies are in business to make a profit, and denial of tests they deem unnecessary only increases the bottom line for their stockholders and their CEOs. The Bible says that people perish for lack of knowledge and understanding (Hosea 4:6). How this rings true in health care, when the patient and consumer doesn't really understand how health insurance works and how profits are generated and what they're giving up when they purchase an advantage plan or an HMO type insurance policy or even a plan with a limited "provider network."

Chapter 11

THE COVID DEBACLE AND THE MEDICAL MAFIA

The COVID pandemic should have been first battled at the primary care and community health level. This did not happen, because the emphasis on medical care in the US is at the hospital and institutional level for many of the reasons previously discussed in this book. The medical-industrial complex has not fully valued or supported primary care, and what should be the foundation of our health care system has further eroded over the past few decades. Now the lack of effective primary care is at least partially responsible for the US paying twice as much for health care as the next country in the developed world. This has caused the overall health of our country to fall to the ranking of thirty-seventh worldwide. Fix primary care, and you reform our broken and dysfunctional health care system. Membership medicine is a proven solution to primary care transformation, and transforming primary care is the key to health care reform.

Never in history has a pandemic or health crisis been so removed from the doctor-patient relationship and physician leadership. In this case, it's been completely taken over by politics, which, in our country, is too often equated with desire for power and control. In all my years as a pharmacologist, researcher, and physician, now spanning five decades, I have never seen so much pressure and lack of rational and scientific thinking and conflicting information surrounding the question of off label use of existing generic medications. This is made especially evident by the fact that no existing drugs were approved for early intervention of COVID, a potentially deadly disease. The most common thing I hear from my patients and friends is that they don't know what to believe anymore. The public is not as stupid as many politicians think. They can often detect lies and half-truths and self-serving decisions.

In November 24, 2020, Joseph A. Ladapo, MD, wrote an opinion column for the *Wall Street Journal* entitled, "Too Much Caution Is Killing COVID Patients." Dr. Ladapo points out that there is a better way to deal with the pandemic than by politicians restricting our liberties and crippling businesses and our economy which prolonged business shutdowns to try and prevent spread of the virus. He points out that too many doctors have interpreted the term "evidence-based medicine" to mean that the evidence for a treatment must be certain and definitive before it can be given to patients. Because accusing a physician of not being "evidence based" can be career-damaging, fear of straying from the pack has prevailed, so inertia and inaction have gained a foothold amid uncertainty about COVID-19 treatments. He goes on to point out that requiring a high degree of certainty during a crisis may elevate the augustness of medical organizations and appease the sensibilities of medical professionals, but it does nothing for patients who desperately need help.

This stigma and even potential legal actions in the US against doctors prescribing older generic drugs in an off-label use, such as hydroxychloroquine and ivermectin, in prevention and early treatment of COVID was effectively stifled. In the face of evidence suggesting the successful use of these older generic drugs, both in the US and worldwide, this hard-line restrictive action in the US may have contributed to many avoidable deaths and hospitalizations during the COVID pandemic, where early intervention and treatment was much needed. Under the leadership of President Trump, some states were given stockpiles of hydroxychloroquine, while others, like Oklahoma, spent $20 million to purchase this cheap generic drug, which went completely wasted due to politics and government restrictions imposed by the FDA. Why was a drug that has been used safely for over 60 years worldwide in the prevention and treatment of malaria restricted from use early and in the outpatient setting for COVID, when there were no other alternatives available. The FDA stated it should only be used in hospitalized patients and then only if they were enrolled in a clinical trial due to the concern for the development of a serious heart arrythmia. The experience and the data worldwide suggested that this medication worked best in the early phase of the disease, not after the hyperinflammatory response had manifested that made so many seriously ill, requiring a ventilator, and carried a high rate of mortality.

United States government agencies have sought to ban doctors from prescribing it outside the hospital setting, and the FDA specifically has placed severe restrictions on its use to treat COVID-19 infections due to serious and life-threatening heart arrythmias, even though it has been used worldwide in millions of patients for decades for the prevention and treatment of malaria without such serious warning. Ironically, it's been used as a standard of care in the treatment of rheumatoid arthritis and in lupus erythematous for many years, although as an off-label treatment, since it has never been tested and approved for either by the FDA. In my view, this is a failure of the NIH, FDA, CDC, state governors, and the medical-industrial complex in general to recognize that COVID-19 infections should first be fought at the primary care level. This decision like all medical decisions should be left to the doctor and patient, after they discuss the risks versus the potential benefits.

This lack of value and support for primary care by Medicare and commercial insurance is demonstrated in the fact that only 4.67 percent of commercial insurance dollars was spent on primary care in 2019. The results have been no surprise to me. There was little support or emphasis given to battling the pandemic on an outpatient basis, but several potentially useful off-label medications were restricted, and nothing was provided to the primary care physician to treat their COVID patients, other than the advice that patients remain in isolation at home and get "supportive therapy." What would have been the harm in prescribing these off-label medications to selected patients with acute COVID infections in hopes of preventing serious illness and even death in so many in our country. It seems unethical and immoral when there was no other outpatient alternative for most of 2020. Again, this is an example of interference with the sacred doctor-patient relationship.

But to the medical-industrial complex, the pathway through evidence-based, prospective, randomized, and controlled clinical trials was the only acceptable course. Unfortunately, the only studies that fit into this category were done in very sick, hospitalized patients, and the methodology among this handful of studies was heterogeneous in my opinion. The term "medical mafia" might seem harsh to some, but one of the definitions of mafia is a closed group of people in a particular field, having a controlling influence. The word seems appropriate in this case. In some ways we can use the medical-industrial complex and the "medical mafia" synonymously.

The decision of closing our economy so people could sheltering at home for months has devasted many of our small businesses and caused millions of our citizens to become unemployed, despite the federal government turning up the printing press for more US dollars, adding to our national debt, which is $28 trillion and growing at the writing of this book. The federal government is the only entity in the US that can habitually spend money it doesn't have and get away with it. Everyone else would be in bankruptcy court and starting over. We, as citizens, again need a constitutional amendment for a balanced federal government budget and term limitation on Congress.

Doctors and those in the public who think critically must ask why there's been such a bias toward an older generic drug called hydroxychloroquine, which has previously been deemed safe. Could it have anything to do with the fact that there's not nearly as much money to be made with the use of this drug as with the use of newer, patented, expensive therapeutics and vaccines? Did it have anything to do with the "Trump derangement syndrome," since he supported the use of the drug both to treat and prevent COVID and admitted he took it himself? Why did certain physicians and scientists in authority insist on looking only at prospective randomized trials, which, at the time of writing this book, did not include early treatment in the outpatient setting? Also, the methodology of those six studies was complex and done in the late, hospitalized stage of the disease. Why did they refuse to consider the large amount of clinical experience and evidence documented in the US and worldwide on the off-label use of medications to treat COVID?

Their decision to block physicians from exercising their right to use medications off-label in the treatment of COVID may have cost hundreds of thousands of lives in the US alone. By February 2021, more than a year after the start of the pandemic, there were over 27 million COVID-19 cases in the US and about 485,500 related deaths, according to Johns Hopkins. Do you appreciate my point that tremendous consequences can occur when politicians interfere with the sacred doctor-patient relationship? Evidence-based medicine was never meant to dominate or tyrannize the physician but to compliment the clinical expertise of the physician as he or she treated the individual patient within the context of the patient's value system and wishes and evaluated the severity of the potential outcomes. The drug was relatively cheap, widely available, and historically safe. What was the harm in using it in higher risk patients as we waited for more effective treatments to become available? The bigger question we must ask is why was it so severely restricted? Drugs are used off-label every day by physicians. Maybe time will tell.

Some doctors argue that in lower doses and for shorter durations of treatment, the drug is even safe enough to be available over the counter. The FDA removed its emergency use authorization for the prescribing of hydroxychloroquine due to a supposed lack of efficacy and the risk of serious heart arrythmias. This put a wall up between pharmacies and patients so that the patients' only way of receiving hydroxychloroquine would be to be sick enough to be admitted to a hospital and the hospital was running an ongoing clinical trial. As one of my patients, who is a critical care nurse at our local hospital told me recently, "We saw promising results with the medication, but it's no longer prescribed, and we don't know why." One of the mechanisms of action of the medication against COVID might be its anti-inflammatory effects. It should be initiated early in the course of the disease, before the "cytokine storm" occurs. It is this hyperinflammatory reaction the virus can cause in some patients with COVID infections that cause them to become seriously ill, go into multi-organ failure, and be at a high risk for dying.

I believe the decline in effective primary care and community health in the US, which has taken place over many decades, significantly contributed to the high morbidity and mortality rate of this awful viral infectious disease. The medical mafia's unwillingness to consider the whole of the evidence and the valuable clinical experience of doctors, in the US and other countries, doesn't seem reasonable. They've effectively removed the one medication that could potentially save lives. Years of gutting out the remnant of primary care physicians and community health in the US, severely limited our ability to treat COVID patients on the outpatient basis. If more value and resources had been brought to bear years ago to primary care before the pandemic, we likely could have further limited hospitalization and death during the pandemic.

On the other hand, thousands of doctors' offices have closed under the financial stress of COVID due to their limited profit margins and need for high volume of daily patient visits. A survey by the Physicians Foundation estimated that 8 percent of all primary care physician practices in the US, or around sixteen thousand, have permanently closed their offices under the stress of the pandemic. Yet, COVID passes stroke, accidents, and Alzheimer's disease as the third leading cause of deaths in US, only surpassed by cardiovascular and cancer deaths. COVID made 2020 the deadliest year in US history and reached 380,000 COVID related deaths in the US. Among all the nations of the world, the US had the highest number of both COVID infections and COVID deaths in 2020.

I'm a strong advocate of the notion that physicians are more than capable of making the right decisions for treatment. They can do this in concert with their patients and without politicians, government agencies, or guidelines. Nothing should interfere with the doctor-patient relationship or put the doctor at risk for using a treatment or medication off-label in an effort to save lives. The irony of this is that for most of 2020, there was no approved alternative treatment in the early outpatient stage, yet the stakes are so high for severe morbidity and mortality. Clearly the potential benefits far outweigh the risks with use of off-label medications.

Therefore I'm so passionate about helping to grow, stabilize, and improve the effectiveness of primary care through the membership model. Physicians must be in control of the profession of medicine, and the patients well-being should be our primary focus.

In an editorial in *The Hill* entitled "Primary Care Doctors Could Be COVID-19's Next Victim," Dr. Tom Frieden, former director of the CDC under President Obama, points out that thousands of primary care practices saw patients when they first developed symptoms, with few resources and inadequate supplies of protective equipment. He also points out that the COVID-19 pandemic highlighted the value of primary care. Unfortunately, he speculates that up to 60,000 primary care physicians could go out of business without additional help from Congress. He points out that primary care is the small business of health care, and it's not too late to save it. Unfortunately, he and others are proposing a capitated payment model, which doesn't fix the problem this book brings to light—that the family physician needs more resources *and* more time to take care of the patient, both in the office and outside the office.

I do agree with him that all over the world (especially in the US), there is overemphasis on hospital care and underemphasis on primary care, outpatient care, and family medicine. As a result, health care generally is less effective and costs more in the US. You, the patient, will have to be smarter, have more common sense, and invest in your own health to get the increased time, focus, and attention you need and deserve. This can only be realistically provided by a membership primary care physician. You will look back, like so many of our membership patients, and realize it was the best investment you ever made, because when you have your health, you have everything, and when you lose your health, you have nothing.

Chapter 12

BAILEY FAMILY MEDICAL CARE: PROTOTYPE FOR MEMBERSHIP MEDICINE

Dr. Bailey, in my view, represents the doctor of the future and probably the last hope for really dealing with the health care crisis in an effective and brilliant manner.

—Gary S., patient of Dr. Bailey and Bailey Family Medical Care, PC

A patient must have a paradigm shift in thinking about interaction with a membership primary care practice and physician to have a value-based experience. Many patients have never been in a membership medical practice and simply don't fully understand how it works and what value it brings to their health and lives and those of their family. For those who lack experience with this newer and better way of delivering primary care, I wish to provide a detailed orientation as he or she interacts with their new medical clinic staff and their membership doctor going forward. It's worth emphasizing the dos and don'ts for the patient. It's also important to point out how membership care is vastly different from the current, large-volume, fee-for-service, discounted, insurance-base primary care practice.

With all interactions in life, first there's a period of getting to know each other. Then a level of friendship is developed, and out of this relationship, trust and respect develop. Only after this is achieved can successful diagnostic and therapeutic transactions occur. This process is achieved much more quickly if the new patient knows about their membership doctor, his or her educational and personal background, the doctor's strengths, and their uniqueness in their approach to patient care.

A good way for the patient to get knowledgeable is to review the practice website. This is true across all specialties of medicine, but never more important than in the doctor you will be looking to as your primary care physician (PCP).

This is your new medical home. The doctor is the navigator of your health and wellness through an overly expensive, dysfunctional, and inefficient health care system. It will likely be extremely frustrating, impersonal, and lacking in excellence in customer service. An effective membership primary care physician and staff will hold your hand, advise you, and walk you through each step of a specialist's referral, getting testing done, and engaging with the complexities of your local hospital. This is stressful enough for the patient, and for our older patients, everything has become much more demanding and impersonal during the COVID pandemic. This includes the elderly who have been isolated, or anyone who's scheduled for a procedure or operation or is sick enough to require hospitalization. Could we ever have imagined a time when the patient's spouse or next of kin couldn't see them in the hospital or be present to see that their advance directives were followed per the patient's legally expressed wishes.

Your membership primary care physician has intentionally reduced his or her patient panel size, often down to only 10 percent of the patient panels that existed before converting to a membership practice (i.e., from several thousands to several hundreds).

This is a game changer for you as the patient. By becoming a member in a primary care membership practice, you have moved away from being just a number and experiencing a seven-minute doctor appointment. You have also decreased the chances that prescribed physician orders and services will be delayed and/or carried out in an inefficient manner that are often experienced in an traditional primary care practice. Traditionally, medicine is practiced in a highly complex system carried out by an often-incompetent medical office staff that frequently turns over, and they often don't have the same commitment to you as your physician. A doctor under this level of stress may already be burned out from the imposed bureaucracy, heavy regulations, and mounds of documentation required by the federal government and the commercial health insurance companies. But the razor's edge finances that a primary care physician lives with day in and day out, is made much worse by not seeing large numbers of patients in the office daily. This loss of patient revenue becomes the most expensive item when a doctor takes a family vacation or a continuing medical education trip.

This means that in a membership practice, you're getting time, focus, and attention at levels of ten to a hundred times greater than you had in your previous high-volume, traditional primary care practices. Remember, there is a lot of time spent by the physician and staff that's behind the scenes—refilling your scripts, researching, and answering your requests and questions, calling for office notes, test results, scheduling, and clarifying your specialist appointments, including coordinating your care to the emergency room and hospital admissions, all in a timely manner.

Although, as spelled out in this book, there are numerous direct and indirect benefits for the cost of a gourmet cup of coffee daily, the greatest benefit is that your membership payment allows the doctor to go down to 200 to 500 active patients, so you receive his or her full focus and attention on your journey of health and wellness.

Bailey Family Medical Care, PC, is a prototype for an expanded service membership family medicine practice. "A Whole Person Approach for the Whole Family" has been our tag line for the practice for 18 years. I have personalized the way I practice and the way I deliver medicine to my patients, specializing in micronutrient therapy and the BaleDoneen Method, in order to prevent diseases and/or detect them early by identifying their root causes and fashioning life style modifications before the disease process becomes chronic, longstanding, and irreversible. This personalized health care model is a revolutionary model of medical practice that puts you, the patient, at the center of the health care experience, utilizing the most advanced technology to both prevent and reverse disease processes early before it leads to increased morbidity and mortality.

Philosophy of Care

Bailey Family Medical Care, PC, has a mission of putting the patient first, from the time you first step into the office. Once you become a member-patient, you're entitled to all the continued care provided to you inside and outside the office setting, meeting you the patient along the way in your day-to-day activities, wherever you are and whenever you need care or consultation. I and my team provide detailed and coordinated care in a loving fashion. We always have time for your questions and concerns.

We listen carefully to each and every question and concern our patients have and incorporate my expertise, careful evaluation of the evidence in the medical literature, and consider you the patient's value system in making an accurate diagnosis and in fashioning an effective, individualized treatment plan, which includes lifestyle changes and nutrition and medical-grade nutritional supplements, before turning to medications and surgery.

What Is Membership Medicine?

Patients pay an annual fee to Bailey Family Medical Care in return for program services, which includes:

- An annual private checkup, regardless of medical condition or necessity
- Enhanced health guidance
- Electronic communication connection with your physician regarding your health information or data
- Assistance with using that data more effectively toward achieving health goals identified based on your annual private checkup

In addition to program services, there are incidental conveniences associated with program membership. I as your primary care physician am no longer dependent on plan-controlled care, so your office visits are unhurried. With the private checkup implementation, you'll enjoy same day/next day communication. You'll also have easy, direct communication with Bailey Family Medical Care via a phone call to the front office during business hours. You'll be able to access me directly through a patient portal, phone messages, emails, or text for questions related to health care education, patient health care support, diet, nutrition, and fitness education goals not covered by your plan. These benefits are available because I as your physician have detached from dependence on time-restricted plan reimbursements and I am enabled by your private fee investment in your health.

Benefits of Membership?

An annual, regardless of medical condition or necessity, medical examination, or physical checkup ("private checkup")

Enhanced health guidance and electronic communication connection with me as your physician regarding your patient health information or data

Assistance with using that data more effectively toward achieving health goals, identified during the annual private checkup

Also, because of me having a smaller patient panel, in addition to the program services, you as the patient will experience:

- Increased access, including having my cell phone number for text or call for emergencies after hours or on weekends
- Same-day or next-day appointments
- Minimal time in the check-in room
- Appointments routinely start on time
- Health care support regarding diet, nutrition, and fitness goals that may not be covered by your health care plan
- Complementary and alternative medicine (CAM) programs offered by me and my team as an independent integrated membership family medicine physician

As a potential new member of the practice, I encourage you to take the time to read and study the printed and electronic material on me and our membership practice. Most membership primary care physicians will have a well-developed, informative website and brochure. See www.baileyfamilymedicalcare.com for a broad array of information on me and my practice. It even includes a copy of my patient membership contract, my complete academic curriculum vitae for review, our mission statement, patient reviews, and several videos of me explaining my background and why I chose family medicine and specialized programs I offer. There's also information about the BaleDoneen Method, our team, contact information, a list of services I provide, and even a direct link with our patient portal once you're established as a member. Out of all of this, you should be able to get a good idea of the ethos of the practice and determine from your prospective as a patient if this is the type of experience you're seeking from your membership doctor and practice, and your new medical home.

Most membership primary care physicians, including me, are looking for patients to do their due diligence and commit to the annual membership because we're looking for long-term relationships to maximize the benefits of the program for health and wellness. I as the doctor and my staff put an enormous amount of time and effort into often gathering hundreds of pages of old medical records, studying them, and indexing them to your new electronic medical record. This is all done before your first appointment. If you request it, you can have a meet-and-greet appointment prior to the first appointment with me, so you'll know exactly what you're investing in. Patients who neglect to take the time to go through these steps often are not just sampling the waters, but potentially wasting their time and that of the doctor and staff in getting you the patient properly established.

Another approach to take in evaluating your new membership physician is to review his or her education, training, and life experience, because they can vary dramatically. A good place to start is to review the doctors complete curriculum vitae. There are two major things that distinguish me from most other primary care physicians. First, I hold the doctor of pharmacy (PharmD) degree and completed the most hands-on, patient-oriented, hospital-based, two-year clinical pharmacy residency training program at the University of Kentucky teaching hospital, in Lexington, Kentucky. In this two-year post-PharmD residency, I worked over a hundred hours per week, working many night shifts as the only pharmacist running the central pharmacy in a 450-bed hospital. My duties included working with all the doctors and nurses in direct patient care and staffing all codes in the hospital and emergency room in preparing intravenous medications from the crash cart. This experience provided me with a level of patient care activity that better prepared me for patient care in my medical training. Second, I spent nearly ten years on the full-time medical faculty of surgery and as Director of Surgical Research at Creighton University, in Omaha, Nebraska, before going to medical school. After medical school and family medicine residency training, I was appointed to the full-time faculty of Mayo Medical School in family medicine and as the Director of Research for Family Medicine at Mayo Clinic, Scottsdale.

These two different careers prior to practicing family medicine in private practice provided me with the background to help my patients in all areas of medicine and surgery. It gave me the broad background and exposure in medicine and surgery a doctor needs to practice the full spectrum of family medicine in this high tech medical and research environment. Although doctors, like others online, are occasionally vulnerable to a bad review due to a disgruntled former employee or a patient whose expectations were not met, I look at the overall reviews and whether or not they're favorable overall. Did the patient comments help you to learn more about your new doctor?

A word of caution: be careful when you see large numbers of reviews and they're all of the highest levels. This may indicate that the doctor utilized commercial resources to actively solicit and front load them, rather than depend on the motivated patient to spontaneously make the reviews. This second approach can take many more years for the doctor to develop adequate reviews, but for me they seem more genuine, and patient driven.

Time with the doctor and his or her staff is the most valuable and rarest commodity in the traditional primary care practice, but it can become a problem if the membership patient doesn't realize that their appointment time, although incredibly generous, is not unlimited. Nor should the patient chronically be late or no show their appointments. The membership doctor has moved from seeing twenty to thirty or more patients in a day to less than ten, so these appointment times are precious. Most are running a hybrid practice, with income coming from both the annual membership fee and in office and telemedicine visits that are reimbursed at a deeply discounted rate by Medicare and commercial insurances. Both these revenue streams are often needed financially to run a practice on ten percent of the doctor's previous patient panel size and at the sparse reimbursement levels for primary care combined with the high overhead of a primary care physician, often eighty percent higher. It's interesting to me that ninety percent of membership doctors say they don't have enough patients in their panels. So, one of the best blessings a patient can provide for their membership doctor is refer a family member or friend who they feel will be a good fit to the practice.

Personally, I schedule two hours for new patients and executive physicals, and I review all active medical problems, extensive laboratory tests, and often other testing. I schedule up to one hour for all other appointments. This usually allows more than enough time to handle all the issues that are scheduled or that arise at the visit. Due to Medicare, commercial insurance requirements, and liability issues, part of this time is needed to document all the elements of the visit. This also allows time for expanded face-to-face time with the doctor, which is not available in a traditional practice.

Your membership primary care physician is most interested in making an early and correct diagnosis and providing effective treatment and prevention strategies. Doctors know that patient education is causally linked to patient compliance. Remember, your doctor is handling multiple other duties during the workday, beyond the in-office patient visits, which include patient emergencies, refilling prescriptions, reviewing test results, reviewing other doctor notes, speaking directly with other doctors, and answering patients calls and various requests that come up each day. Keep in mind that the volume and extent of medical work and documentation in a membership practice increases, rather than decreases, as more services are provided outside the office setting and the doctor is spending more time and attention on a smaller number of patients. The COVID pandemic has intensified these out-of-office patient care activities, and I estimate it has increased my patient care workload by one third. Remember that you want your doctor to be a lifelong learner and to take care of his/her family and this means they may not always be available to see you in the office, but with smart phones, the internet, patient electronic portals, telemedicine audio and video appointments, you membership primary care doctor is always available to connect with you for more urgent health needs and concerns even when he/she is attending a medical course or taking care of their own family.

Patients can help the doctor to be most efficient with their appointment time with the patient in office by coming prepared with a list of questions or concerns they would like to cover in the visit, and providing that list to the medical assistant at the time of check in. It can also be sent ahead of the visit on the patient portal, as some of our patients like to do. In a membership practice, the doctor and staff have carefully prejudged the time they will likely need. The appointment time is never shortened but often lengthened to accommodate the patient and minimize any wait time of the next patient. Therefore, we no longer call it the waiting room but rather the check in lobby.

I hope I have convinced you that a membership primary care physician is the most important member of your health care team. Ideally, you want an independent, personal, caring, compassionate, scientifically trained, integrated primary care physician who has the necessary time to take care of you and coordinate your health care experience and be the custodian of your entire medical record and the navigator of your health care experience and wellness journey.

Even if you can find a primary care physician with some or all of these qualities, under the current reimbursement system, they simply won't have enough time to do the job right, because the fully functioning primary care physician has not been valued or supported by the government and third-party payers, or, for that matter, the medical-industrial complex. Paying primary care physicians only a small fraction earned by their specialist colleagues has forced them to live on a razor's edge of profitability and see just as many patients in their office as is humanly possible. It is like the gerbil on the wheel. The wheel keeps going faster and faster.

The problem we have going forward with traditional primary care is that there simply isn't enough money to reimburse primary care physicians what they should be paid to do the job correctly. The extra money has been paid out to the hospitals, pharmaceutical companies, specialists, and procedures instead of for the cognitive and diagnostic and educational work and coordination that one would expect form their primary care doctor. This is because we, as a society, are dealing with a deficit of $28 trillion, and it's still growing.

We have a severe shortage of primary care physicians. This shortage is being filled by nurse practitioners and physician assistants and protocol medicine and soon artificial intelligence. Many of our brightest and best medical students want to go into family medicine but can't afford too financially. They are also discouraged when they see the scope of family medicine narrowed and the lack of respect for their specialty of family medicine. In addition, they don't make enough income to pay off their large educational debt or to justify their long hours of work and the sacrifices of their families. In specialty medicine, they're paid more respect, reimbursed at a much higher rate, and have a more balanced life for their family and their own mental health. The membership model really is a win-win-win situation—for the patient, the doctor, and our broken health care system. I think this is the key to overall health care reform.

If you have read this book to the end, I congratulate you, because you're interested in finding the most effective pathway to improved health, and you're likely an individual who desires to see health care in the US reformed so that it's less costly, less dysfunctional, better coordinated, and helps to move the US to the top rather than the bottom of health among all the developed nations.

Rather than move to socialized medicine, as represented in Obamacare or Medicare for all, we're proposing a healthy, capitalist approach to empower you, the user, in the most major and effective reform of primary care in our nation's modern history. You might find it interesting that membership primary care is so valuable to me and my family personally that we too invest with a membership primary care doctor. I believe it's one of the smartest and most valuable financial investments I've made. It increases our odds of living longer, being healthier, and avoiding a catastrophic financial health crisis.

As one of my patients said, her relative told her she should never let her membership with Dr. Bailey expire, because it's worth every penny. I hope you'll join the ever-growing ranks of us who are fortunate enough to have a membership primary care physician who genuinely cares for us and walks alongside us in our life's journey of health, healing, and wholeness. May God bless you and your family, and may you know His love and concern for you and all that affects your life and well-being, in your body, mind, and spirit. To your health. Dr. Bailey

Acknowledgements

I respectfully acknowledge the life and memory of Dr. C. C. Wanamaker (1923–1996), a great family physician role model to me and to thousands in the cities of Charleston and North Charleston, South Carolina. He was greatly admired and loved by his patients and the citizens of North Charleston, and greatly respected by his specialty colleagues in Charleston and by the leaders on the Charleston County Council, where he served for many years.

Dr. Wannamaker was fiercely independent and outspoken but kind. Doc had served as a family doctor in North Charleston for forty-two years and as an elected representative of Charleston County for thirty-two years. Dr. Charlie put his patients, and only his patients, first. I often saw his office packed with all sorts of patients, from the well to the sick, and even some injured. The patients never complained when they had to wait up to four hours or even longer to see him. They were just thankful that Dr. Wannamaker was their personal physician, and he would stay until everyone was seen.

Everyone knew that Dr. Wannamaker was a great diagnostician who worked harder, was smarter, but made a lot less money than the specialty colleagues he referred his patients to, mostly in downtown Charleston, very much a town-and-gown medical society. We knew his motives were pure and his patients were his highest priority. Unlike the sometimes large egos and pretense of the specialists, Dr. Charlie did not have to pretend; he was smart, confident, dedicated, and focused on helping us get well. He was that old-fashion kind of country doctor that still made house calls. Without experiencing his model of care and dedication, I would not have made pharmacy and medicine my career choice. Pharmacy, for me, was a career choice, but later in life, it became clear that medicine would be a lifestyle choice. It's underappreciated today that physicians make a tremendous sacrifice for their patients if they care and have righteous motives.

I also want to acknowledge my brilliant and talented wife, Johanna Sue Bailey, whose first instincts were right when a "prophet" asked her if she had considered the doctor in her church for a husband. She said, "He's had his head in his books way too long." But she, like I, left some very precious family behind for a season, to pursue the "City of God," as Abraham did, as is written about in Genesis. We relocated to Scottsdale, AZ, in 1999 to plant a nondenominational Christian church, and we watched the water level of God rise in the greater Phoenix area.

God rewarded us with each other, a marriage arranged, you might say, by our Heavenly Father. We were given so many wonderful opportunities through the years to assist the pastor of our church and his family and many others in the church. We helped our community by providing medical care and Christian service. We headed up the personal prophetic prayer for the church congregants for many years. Johanna came to work by my side in private practice (Bailey Family Medical Care, PC, www.baileyfamilymedicalcare.com) in 2003 and has been key to our success, both in independent practice and, later, converting to a membership-based medical practice. She has served as our office manager and in-patient educator, and together we've committed ourselves to lifelong learning and to seeing justice and righteousness be restored to our great profession of medicine;

to the educational system; and to our local, state, and federal government. We live in a time when this has never been needed as much as it is now. At times it seems as if our great country has lost its way, but our trust is in the Lord (Isa. 59:4–8).

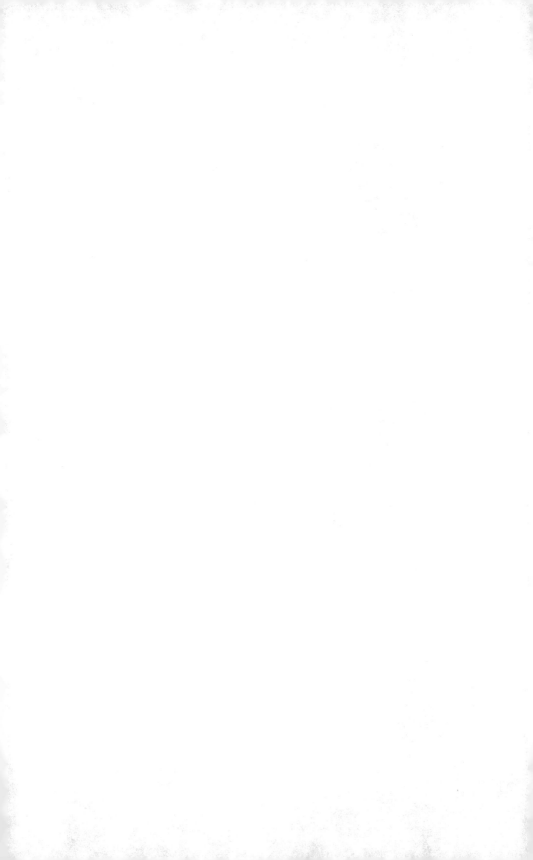

Bibliography

Membership Primary Care

Bruno, Janet. *Creating Patients for Life.* Fountain Hills: Bruno Press, 2012.

Tetreault, Michael, Catherine Sykes. *The Doctor's Expanded Guide to Concierge Medicine.* Alpharetta: Elite MD Publishing, 2020.

Tetreault, Michael. *Branding Concierge Medicine.* Alpharetta: Elite MD Publishing, 2012.

Tetreault, Michael. *The Marketing M.D.* Alpharetta: Docpreneur Press, 2015.

Family Medicine Reform

"AAFP Gives Administration Formula for Saving Primary Care." www.aafp.org/news. (May 11, 2020).

Sur, Roger L, Philipp Dahm. "History of Evidence-Based Medicine." *Indian J Urol* 27(4) 2011: 487-89.

Starfield, Barbara. "Commentary on Regular Primary Care Lowers Hospitalization and Mortality in Seniors with Chronic Respiratory Disease." *J Gen Intern Med* 25(8) 2010:758-59.

Starfield, Barbara, Leiyu Shi, James Macinko. "Primary Care Contribution to Health Systems and Health." *Milbank Q* 83(8) 2005:457-502.

Webb, Nicholas J. *The Cost of Being Sick: A Prevention Initiative*. Orem: Sound Concepts, Inc., 2010.

Integrated Primary Care

Balch, Phyllis A. *Prescription for Nutritional Healing*. New York: Avery, 2006.

Bland, Jeffrey, Thomas G. Guilliams. "Cardiovascular Disease: New Clinical Options for Expanding the Therapeutic Target" Part 1 and Part 2. *Lifestyle Resource Center Matrix Blog. Woodstock: 2018.*

Contreras, Francisco, and Daniel E. Kennedy. *Fighting Cancer 20 Different Ways (Preventing it. Reversing it.)*. Lake Mary: Siloam, 2005.

Ghosh, Tarini S, Simone Rampelli, Ian B Jeffery, et al. "Mediterranean Diet Intervention Alters the Gut Microbiome in Older People Reducing Frailty and Improving Health Status: The NU-AGE 1-Year Dietary Intervention Across Five European Countries." *Gut* 69(7) 2020: 1218-1228.

Gittleman, Ann Louis. *Fat Flush for Life: The Year-Round Super Detox Plan to Boost Your Metabolism and Keep the Weight Off Permanently*. Cambridge: First Da Capo Press, 2010.

Guilliams, Thomas G. *Supplementing Dietary Nutrients: A Guide for Healthcare Professionals Second Edition*. Stevens Point: Point Institute, 2020.

Guilliams, Thomas G and Roni Enten. *The Original Prescription: How the Latest Scientific Discoveries Can Help You Leverage the Power of Lifestyle Medicine.* Stevens Point, Point Institute, 2012.

Hyman, Mark. *The Blood Sugar Solution: The ultra-Healthy Program for Losing Weight, Preventing Disease, and feeling Great Now!* New York: Little, Brown and Company, 2012.

Hyman, Mark. *Eat Fat, Get Thin: Why the Fat We Eat is the Key to Sustained Weight Loss and Vibrant Health.* New York: Little, Brown and Company, 2016.

Kaats, Gilbert R. *Restructuring Body Composition: How the kind, not the amount, of weight loss defines a pathway to optimal health.* Dallas: Taylor Publishing Company, 2008.

Mathuna, Donal O, Walt Larimore. *Alternative Medicine: The Christian Handbook.* Grand Rapids: Zondervan Publishing House, 2001.

Mugent, Steve. *How to Survive on a Toxic Planet.* Davao City, Philippines: Alethia Corporation, 2004.

Thompson, Rob. *Glycemic Load Diet.* New York: McGraw-Hill, 2006.

The BaleDoneen Method

Bale, Brad F, Amy L Doneen, Lisa Collier Cool. *Beat the Heart Attack Gene: The Revolutionary Plan to Prevent Heart Disease, Stroke, and Diabetes.* Nashville: Turner Publishing, 2014.

Bale, Brad F, Amy L Doneen, Ross Drueding, et al. "Aggressive Risk Factor Modification in Patients with Sub-Clinical Atherosclerosis Reduces Plaque Burden and regresses Carotid Artery Wall Thickness." *Atherosclerosis* 7(3): 2006, 161.

Cheng, Henry G, Birju S Patel, Seth S Martin, et al. "Effect of Comprehensive Cardiovascular Disease Risk Management on Longitudinal Changes in Carotid Artery Intima-Media Thickness in a Community-Based Prevention Clinic." *Arch Med Sci* 12(4): 2016, 728-735.

Doneen, Amy L and Brad F Bale. "Carotid Intima-Media Thickness Testing as an Asymptomatic Cardiovascular Disease Identifier and Method for Making Therapeutic Decisions." *Postgrad Med* 125(2): 2013, 108-122.

Feng, Du, M Christina Esperat, Amy L Doneen, et al. " Eight-year Outcomes of a Program for Early Prevention of Cardiovascular Events: A Growth-Curve Analysis." *J Cardiovasc Nurs* 30(4): 2015, 281-91.

Nutritional Supplements

Blumberg, Jeffrey B, Balz Frei, Victor L Fulgoni, et al. "Vitamin and Mineral Intake is Inadequate for Most Americans: What Should We Advise Patients About Supplements?" *J Fam Pract* 65(9 suppl): 2016, 1-8.

Houston, Mark K. "The Role of Cellular Micronutrients Analysis, Nutraceuticals, Vitamins, Antioxidants, and Minerals in the Prevention and Treatment of Hypertension and Cardiovascular Disease." *Ther Adv Cardiovasc Dis* 0 (0):2010, 1-19.

Morris, Martha K, Christine C Tangney. "A Potential Design Flaw of Randomized Trials of Vitamin Supplements." *JAMA* 305(13):2011, 1348-1349.

Murray, Robert K, Daryl K Granner, Victor W Rodwell. "Glycoproteins" In Harper's Illustrated Biochemistry 27th

Edition Edited by Victor W Rodwell, Daryl K Granner, Peter A Mayes, et al.523-544. New York: McGraw Hill Lange, 2006.

Faith and Medicine

Brand, Paul and Philip Yancey. *Fearfully and Wonderfully Made.* Grand Rapids: Zondervan Publishing House, 1980.

Grant, Wilson W. "The Two Diagnoses." *Today's Christian Doctor.* Fall of 2017.

Levin, Jeff. "Partnerships Between the Faith-Based and medical Sectors: Implications for Preventative medicine and Public Health." *Prev Med Rev* 4: 2016, 344-50.

Reed, William S. *Surgery of the Soul: healing the Whole Person Spirit, Mind, and Body.* Tampa: Christian Medical Foundation, International, Inc., 1995.

Post, Stephen G, Christina M Puchalski, David B Larson. "Physicians and Patients Spirituality: Professional Boundaries, Competency and Ethics. *Ann Int med* 132(7): 2020, 578-583.

Health Insurance

Cogan, John F, Rlenn Hubbard, Daniel P Kesler. *Healthy, Wealthy, and Wise.* Jackson: AEI Press, 2005.

Hopper, Robert and Debra Hopper. *Healthcare Happily Ever After: A Friendly Little Tale of the Health Savings Account and How It Won the Heart of a Nation.* Overland Park: A.D. Banker and Company, L.L.C., 2007.

McCaughey, Betsy. *Beating Obamacare: Your Handbook for Surviving the New Health Care Law.* Washington: Regnery Publishing, Inc., 2013.

Pilzer, Paul Z. *The New Health Insurance Solution: How to Get Cheaper, Better Coverage Without a Traditional Employer Plan.* Hoboken: John Wiley and Sons, Inc., 2005.

Tate, Nick J. *ObamaCare Survival Guide: The Affordable Care Act and What It means for You and Your Healthcare.* West Palm Beach: Humanix Books, 2012.

The COVID-19 Pandemic

Al-Bari, Abdul A. "Chloroquine Analogues in Drug Discovery: New Directions of Uses, mechanisms of Actions and Toxic Manifestations from Malaria to Multifarious Diseases." *J Antimicrob Chemother* 70(6) 2015: 1608-21.

Bale, Brad F, Amy L Doneen, Thomas Hight, et al. "Enhancement of Innate Immunity to COVID-19 with Natural Measures." *Immunome Res* 16(3): 2020, 1-4.

"FDA Cautions Against Use of Hydroxychloroquine or Chloroquine for COVID-19 Outside of the Hospital Setting or a Clinical Trial Due to Risk of Heart Rhythm Problems" FDA Drug Safety Communication, US food and Drug Administration, April 24, 2020, Updated June 15, 2020.

Gautret, Philippe, Jean-Christophe Lagier, Philippe Parola, et al. Hydroxychloroquine and Azithromycin as a Treatment of COVID-19: Results of an Open-Label non-Randomized Clinical Trial." *Int J Antimicrob Agents* 56(1): 2020, 106949.

Huang, Chaolin, Yeming Wang, Xingwang Li, et al. "Clinical Features of Patients Infected with 2019 Novel Coronavirus in Wuhan, China." *The Lancet* 395 (10223): Feb 15, 2020, 497-506.

Ladapo, Joseph A "Too Much Caution is Killing COVID Patients." *WSJ*: Nov 24, 2020.

Mega, Teshale A, Temesgen M Feyissa, Dula D Bosho, et al. "The Outcome of Hydroxychloroquine in Patients Treated for COVID-19: Systematic Review and Metanalysis." *Can Respir J* 2020: 4312519 (published on-line Oct 13, 2020).

Sun, JingKang, YuTing Chen, XiuDe Fan, et al. "Advances in the Use of Chloroquine and Hydroxychloroquine for the Treatment of COVID-19." *Postgrad Med* 132(7): Jun 21, 2020, 604-613.

About the Author

Dr. Bailey is a recognized thought leader in family medicine, primary care, and clinical pharmacy. During his formative years, Dr. Bailey was motivated and inspired to enter the medical field and family medicine by his medical role model, Dr. C. C. Wannamaker, an outstanding family physician in North Charleston, South Carolina, in the 1960s and 1970s. He was also called to full-time Christian ministry as a young boy and initially envisioned himself going to seminary to become an ordained Methodist minister in South Carolina, his home state. But God had different plans. As they say, God works in mysterious ways. He was greatly influenced by the strong Methodist pastors he interacted with in the 1960s and '70s, including Oral Roberts, who was part of the Methodist Church during this time. Ironically, thirty years later Dr. Bailey was trained in a family medicine residency in Tulsa, OK, called In His Image, which originated as the official Family Medicine Residency Program of Oral Roberts University School of Medicine, from the late 1970s to the late '80s.

Dr. Bailey has spent the last four decades in the medical field and the last twenty-five years as a practicing family Christian physician. He has personally experienced the takeover of the medical field by the federal and state governments, for-profit health insurance companies, and large and powerful for profit and non-profit hospitals and medical systems.

He has observed, first-hand, how family medicine has been underutilized, underappreciated, and underfunded to the detriment of all patients and of health care in general. He believes that reform and full support of family medicine and primary care is the key in reforming our broken and dysfunctional health care system.

In 2012, out of frustration over not having enough time and resources to take care of his patients the way he knew an independent, integrated family physician should in a unique and excellent way, he converted his large-volume patient practice (over 2,000 patients) to that of a membership model, to the delight of many of his patients.

Dr. Bailey has been in independent, private practice medicine for the past eighteen years and has received numerous patient awards, including Patient Choice Physician Awards, America's Most Compassionate Doctor Awards, Phoenix Magazine Top Doctor Award, Top 10 Family Doctor and Medical Practice in Scottsdale, Arizona, and the NCQA/ADA Physician Diabetic Recognition Program Award. He successfully moved from a tenured and salaried career in academia to creating a prototype model for whole-person medicine of the body, mind, and spirit. His unique approach to patient care and whole-person medicine attracted over six hundred patients from Mayo Clinic, Scottsdale, to follow him to his new community-based practice.

Dr. Bailey is a board-certified family medicine physician and a fellow of the American Academy of Family Physicians. He holds both doctor of medicine and doctor of pharmacy degrees and has done extended residency training in both fields. His background is broad and diverse. Dr. Bailey has served as a tenured associate professor of surgery, family medicine, and pharmacy at Creighton University School of Medicine and as Director of Surgical Research at Creighton University in the 1980s. In addition, he has served as an associate professor of family medicine at Mayo Clinic School of

Medicine and Director of Research for Family Medicine at Mayo Clinic, Scottsdale. He is founder and president of Bailey Family Medical Care, in Scottsdale, Arizona, since 2003 (www.baileyfamilymedicalcare.com) and is a specialist in the BaleDoneen Heart Attack and Stroke Prevention Method. He is an expert in the integration of pharmaceuticals and nutraceuticals in the treatment of his patients.

Dr. Bailey has an illustrious academic career spanning more than forty years and has been awarded numerous large research grants from the National Institutes of Health and the Health Futures Foundation in esophageal disease and left ventricular heart assist devices as a bridge to heart transplant. These grants have totaled more than 1 million dollars on a yearly basis. His research, scholarly work, and publication in peer-reviewed journals, in concert with Dr. Tom R. DeMeester, Chair of Surgery at Creighton University and the Surgical Faculty in the 1980s, resulted in a surgical research program recognized nationally and internationally by numerous chairs of surgery as a model program to facilitate surgical research in their academic centers.

During his time on the faculty at Creighton University, he was awarded twenty-nine research grants and published thirty-seven abstracts, twenty-five scientific manuscripts in peer-reviewed refereed journals, and two book chapters. He has presented sixty-eight scientific presentations and was twice invited to be a guest visiting professor. In private medical practice, he continues to serve on a voluntary basis as associate clinical professor of surgery and family medicine at Creighton University School of Medicine, in Omaha, Nebraska, and Phoenix, Arizona.

Whereas full-time medicine is his vocation, Dr. Bailey's advocation is music. As a trained baritone classical singer, he has had numerous solo performances over the years and was selected as the inaugural baritone soloist for the Charleston Symphony

Chorus. He has performances at the world-renowned Spoleto and Piccolo Festivals, USA, and has sung a principal role in Puccini's *La Boheme*, at the University of Kentucky Opera Series.

Dr. Bailey is a Christian physician and minister and was ordained as a full-time Christian minister of medicine by William Standish Reed, MD, surgeon and family physician, who pioneered the healing of the whole person through the spirit, mind, and body. Dr. Reed was the first physician in the United States to do so. Dr. Reed was deeply influenced by the writings and teachings on whole-person medicine by Swiss family physician and minister Paul Tornier, MD, who has been called the twentieth century's most famous Christian physician.

Dr. Bailey serves as president of a nonprofit organization, Prophet's Reward, Inc., to further positive health care reform in primary care and to advance his Christian ministry, training, and the marriage of faith and medicine. Prophet's Reward is a 501(c)3 nonprofit corporation run out Prayer Mountain, in Moravian Falls, North Carolina, and promotes the opportunity for individuals to pray and meditate on Prayer Mountain. People travel from all over the world to visit, meditate, and pray there. Tax-deductible donations can be made to Prophet's Reward, Inc. and are appreciated, since these donations further the organization's mission. To donate, visit www.prophetsreward.org.

Dr. Bailey has a passion for helping independent primary care physicians convert their practices to a membership primary care practice, and he can be contacted at rbailey@drbaileyclinic.com or at 480- 860-5533 for formal consultation on all aspects of practice conversion.

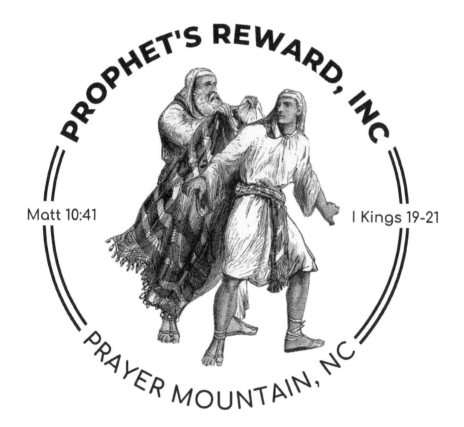

CPSIA information can be obtained
at www.ICGtesting.com
Printed in the USA
BVHW080859120721
611731BV00001B/100